AF660208

The

CHARISMA FACTOR

Leesa Rowland's charisma has led to her success as an author, actress, and animal advocate. The daughter of an artist and college professor, Leesa grew up in Austin, Texas where she learned strong family values and reliance on self-motivation. While in Texas, she studied broadcast journalism and later became a classically trained actress at the world-renowned Stella Adler Studio in Los Angeles. Her acting career includes both television and full-length movie productions.

Beyond her extensive career and credits as a film and television actress, Leesa is the author of the best-selling self-help/motivational book *Discovering the It Factor within You: Developing Your Charismatic Personality*, which was published in 2015. She is also well-known for her work as a philanthropist and animal rights activist. A vegan dedicated to healthy eating, she has been active with the national non-profit organization Last Chance for Animals since 1989 and is the president of the New York non-profit group Animal Ashram, which she founded in 2013.

The CHARISMA FACTOR

Unlock the Secrets of
Magnetic Charm and Personal
Influence in Your Life

LEESA ROWLAND

RUPA

Published by
Rupa Publications India Pvt. Ltd 2024
7/16, Ansari Road, Daryaganj
New Delhi 110002

Sales centres:
Bengaluru Chennai
Hyderabad Jaipur Kathmandu
Kolkata Mumbai Prayagraj

Published in arrangement with Hatherleigh Press

P-ISBN: 978-93-5702-818-9
E-ISBN: 978-93-5702-762-5

First impression 2024

10 9 8 7 6 5 4 3 2 1

Printed in India

Contents

Preface

I was adopted when I was just a few months old by loving parents who had already adopted another daughter at birth. My father, Dr. George Rowland, was a college professor; my mother, Kay, was an extremely talented artist. On the canvas that was my life, these two were the first painters.

The first, but by no means the last. I have such vivid memories of my childhood and the people who shaped it, who showed me love and taught me the important life lessons I've continued to carry on to this day. I went through many personal transformations to get to where I am today, and I am appreciative of the generous help I received along the way. For this reason, I have no doubt I will spend the rest of my life helping others and giving back.

After my parents divorced when I was six years old, my mother, sister, and I moved into my mother's parents' guesthouse on the beach in the resort town of Rockport, Texas. All of a sudden, I had the luxury of having grandparents in my day-to-day life: my grandfather, Jesse M. Davis, had just retired as the head of litigation for Shell Oil Company, while my grandmother, Lavina, would teach me the benefits of organic, unprocessed foods and yoga. They also taught me to respect animals and to treat them like the individual souls they are. These aspects continue to be integral to my life, and have shaped the book that you now hold in your hands.

I am thankful for all the souls I have been fortunate to meet along the way. Some have brought me joy; others have taught me very difficult lessons, but I believe there is something—be it good or bad—that we can learn from everyone. We are all on our own custom-built expeditions, and it is up to us to navigate ourselves through the course our life takes. We are all different, and that is where our strengths lie—we need only learn when and how to put the blinders on and remain true to ourselves.

Throughout my life, I have studied religion, spirituality, yoga, chakras, auras, energy fields, and the supernatural as well. I have always been fascinated with charisma and have researched and studied it for more than twenty years. I also often incorporate practices and techniques that I have learned from method acting studies into my everyday life.

I am, fundamentally, a free spirit. I'm openhearted, nonjudgmental, candid, optimistic and very adventurous. I appreciate that the length of my time on Earth is unknown, so I intend to make the most of it. Mine is a deeply spiritual road, and I try vehemently to live my life in the present moment. While I do believe in an almighty force which I choose to call God, I have always been a firm believer in karma: I believe we reap what we sow and that we are each of us at the reins of our own enlightenment and destiny.

Life is about living well and taking advantage of every single minute we are given. Experience life as it happens, treat every moment as an amazing gift, and you will be well on your way to discovering the extraordinary spark inside yourself, that "It" factor.

I wrote this book to share my story and to help guide others as they embark on their journeys or else come to crossroads of negative or conditioned blockages. I'm sharing the way I navigated through the tough times and how I have maintained the sort of positive outlook that is essential to attaining and retaining a charismatic personality.

And there *have* been tough times in my life—plenty of them, far beyond what I would have ever thought possible. Perhaps my greatest personal struggle has come from my mother's death 15 years ago, something which I still don't have closure for. My mother's significant other at the time (I had moved out of our home at 18 and he moved in with my mother and grandmother shortly afterward) committed suicide by shooting himself several years ago, but not before admitting to family and friends that he had killed my precious mother by poisoning her food. The poison he'd used mimicked the symptoms of a stroke; in fact, that is still listed on her death certificate as the cause of death. There was no autopsy, as he had her cremated the next day.

My mother's tragic death has caused my sister, Karen, and I intense, often debilitating agony. It is one of the deepest, saddest, sharpest, most helpless pains I have ever experienced. And it was a pain that seemed determined to bear yet more hardship. After my mother died, I decided that it was a good time to get to know a group of people who had found me through my father on the internet. They introduced themselves as my long-lost biological cousins, and seemed to make a special effort to reach out quite a bit. My real family, the family who had taken me in and raised me, seemed hurt by the thought that I would give the time of day to anyone who abandoned me as a baby, so I hadn't felt good about really getting to know them while my mother was alive.

Realistically, my loving family thought that, given the abandonment issues I already had, that meeting with my cousins wouldn't be a safe risk for me. They were worried that these "cousins" could be opportunists. What was their real motive to want to get to know me? After I spoke with them the first time, I had this gut feeling that maybe my family was right; they might have gotten in touch with me because I had been in movies, and I was worried that they might just be fame seekers.

But after my mother was killed, I went against my gut feelings and visited these possible birth family cousins at their home in the valley outside of Los Angeles. I thought it was the perfect time to get to know them. They'd continued to reach out and seemed to care about getting to know me, even growing old with me as viable family members. I was a little uncomfortable around them initially—they were nothing like the family I grew up with—but I wanted to give them the unconditional love that my adopted mother had instilled in me. The older female cousin seemed a bit jealous of me, but I have dealt with jealous women my entire life. She occasionally made snide comments about my looks, my acting or charity events I'd attend, but I just shrugged it off and loved her anyway.

When I arrived at their home, I had in my suitcases a lot of newly inherited jewelry, very expensive designer coats and clothes from my mother's estate. Included in this was a very expensive collection of sentimental jewelry and a fur from Vail—brand new with the (extremely expensive) price tag still on it. It was very sentimental to my sister because she'd inherited it from our mother, and the cousins marveled at how beautiful everything was and what great taste my mother had. The older female cousin asked if she could borrow the coat to go to a party the next night. I said okay; she seemed so excited to wear it that I felt good letting her borrow it. All I said was, "Just please pray for my sweet mother's soul when you put it on."

At the time, I was planning on leaving Los Angeles to go to New York and establish an apartment there. The female cousin suggested I keep the jewelry collection in their safe; the coat she would keep the in the closet after the party. I could come back later and pick up everything after I had established my place; that way, nothing would get stolen. I thought to myself what a godsend she was. I'd been given no reason to believe otherwise.

We kept in touch by phone while I was in New York (I was working two jobs by this point). I asked her often if my things were safe and she always reassured me that everything was fine. My concern was understandable; after all, my sister and I still hadn't divided everything up between us by then, so the bulk of the inheritance was being kept in this cousin's safe.

Finally, I found an apartment that I just fell in love with. I called my friends and my cousin to tell them how excited I was; I also let my cousin know that I couldn't wait to ship my storage out from Los Angeles to my new NYC apartment.

As the time to close on my new apartment in New York City grew closer, I was getting more concerned about having my belongings sent out. My friend Ronnie said he would help coordinate it from the Los Angeles side, which gave me a big sense of relief. When I spoke to my cousins, they said to make sure and tell him not to worry, that they would get it for me and put it in their garage. That way, I could go through it and pack it before I shipped it out. They even called me three times in one day just asking for Ronnie's number to coordinate everything with him. It seemed they wanted to call him themselves so that I could just keep working and not be bothered. I thought to myself how lucky I am to have these new, kind, and caring cousins in my life. My fear of abandonment was finally melting away.

I even had a plaque made to give them for Christmas, which read *We may not have grown up together, but we will spend our years growing old together. I thank God for the blessing of you in my life.* I couldn't wait to see them again and get to know them better.

To that end, I canceled the plans I had with my boyfriend and friends for Christmas and New Year's in NYC and left happily to visit my newly-found cousins for the holidays, bringing with me carefully selected presents for all of them. They in turn made plans with Ronnie that he would pick me up and drive me to their house. All I could think was how sweet it was of them to do all this for me. I was beginning to think of this as a family reunion.

When I arrived at their house in the valley, I asked if I could go to the garage and start packing up my belongings. But the female cousin wouldn't take me out to the garage right away; she wanted to wait for her husband for some reason unknown to me. It was their home so, of course, I was respectful and patient. They finally let me take a brief look and I was happy to see the beloved dresser my mother had bought for me was there, as well as one of my favorite framed pictures, designer clothes and my beloved captain's hat. (I'd already picked out the perfect spot for my dresser and other beloved items in my new apartment.)

I couldn't wait to go through everything! It would be just like Christmas. I knew I had lots of jewelry and other sentimental belongings tucked away, as well as my personal photo albums from childhood, the Noah's ark quilt my mother painstakingly made for me as a little girl, and needlepoint items she had won awards for.

As for the cousins, their entire grown family lived in the one house, so I got to see them all in one sitting. They all stayed up late, drinking heavily and celebrating New Year's Eve. Over the course of coordinating things with Ronnie, they'd learned that he was the brother of James Caan and how they really wanted to meet him. I know they were all drunk, talking like that—they were aware that I'd had issues with Jimmy years before, so it hurt my feelings a little. It kind of felt like they were taunting me, but it might have just been alcohol leading them to loosen up a bit too much. Since I was still on New York time (which was 3 hours ahead), I just wanted to get some sleep and wake up early the next day for a possible run or jog.

The next day, I woke up, showered and dressed, to find that everyone was passed out with all their clothes on, lying strung out all over the house. The first one up was one of the older guys. I happily greeted him, "Good morning!"

He immediately started screaming at me that he hated me and wanted me out of his house. Then the woman came in and started screaming with him and told me I had to leave. They screamed and screamed, getting louder and louder. Worse, they wouldn't let me have my belongings, saying that if I didn't leave, they would call the police. I wish *I* had called the police; I would still have all my family heirlooms and wouldn't be writing this.

All of this was more than startling; it felt like the bottom fell out of my gut. I wondered what they might have schemed up as I lay sleeping. The woman said they had been talking while I slept and just decided that I had to leave. I was in such shock; I'd *just* arrived the night before and I had trusted them with everything I had. I couldn't understand what had altered their minds while I was sleeping, but I knew I didn't want to stay anywhere I'm not welcome. The woman barely let me gather anything into my suitcase and drove me to another friend's place who happily took me in for the night so I could change my flight home for the next day.

In the end, I had been conned. Getting my storage from me was a heist—they'd never intended to give it back to me. My con artists "cousins" never answered my calls after that. They'd baited me in, gained my trust, set up the heist and pulled it off. Learn from my mistake: always, always trust your initial gut instincts. I went against mine and paid the price.

It was one of the worst possible scenarios that could have happened when meeting your long-lost biological cousins. I was devastated, in absolute tears for months. I still sometimes cry about it. It shattered my heart into a million little pieces.

I asked Ronnie to see if he could get them to give my belongings back to me, but he only knew them through me and claimed to have had no luck with them, either. He tried; I'll give him that credit. I wish he'd suggested I call the police, but at least he tried to get them to do the right thing.

When I returned home from my traumatic experience, my boyfriend Larry offered to get me an attorney, but I wasn't sure I needed to go that route. In the back of my mind, I really believed these con artists cousins would do the right thing.

I was wrong, heart-breakingly wrong.

I *did* hear from the woman once when she showed up in New York City. She asked if she could meet me, so I said yes and canceled my lunch plans. I thought she was coming to apologize and bring some of my belongings; I met her on the literal street corner. It was so odd: she asked me what I used on my face to keep my skin so soft, and I told her I love coconut oil to remove make-up and use Kinerase cream at night. She asked if we could take a selfie; I obliged, and asked her if she'd brought my mother's coat or any of her jewelry. She said no and took off running.

I still don't understand why she was so adamant on taking a selfie if she doesn't like me. It was very strange. I have not seen these con artists to this day, and I am so thankful to the Lord that I am adopted. I am also thankful beyond words for my *real* family and the values and high moral standards they raised me with. What a beautiful silver lining! God truly does weed out those who are not for you. Of course, my fear of abandonment got worse than you could imagine, but I have been working diligently through my trust issues. In spite of it all, I have, for the most part, managed to keep my optimism alive even during this most suffocating time in my life.

People I know only socially likely assume I don't have a care in the world. Those closest to me know my pain best, while others only know enough of it to ask me on occasion, "Leesa, how do you manage?"

Having been asked that question enough times, I have finally decided to respond. My answer is contained within the book you're now reading.

I manage by constantly evolving and by nurturing what I

have decided to call the "charisma factor" within me. Finding your charisma factor means finding your inherent passion—creating an energy that sets you apart from the crowd and makes you special. This energy is unique to each person and is what entices people to want to be around you. I nurture my sanity, my willpower, and my attitude constantly. It is not always easy and takes constant effort. My heart is still broken, but I refuse to let any situation define me. I refuse to be bitter. I know that every obstacle we encounter is an opportunity for us to grow both personally and spiritually. Opportunity follows struggle.

I don't want this book to be about me, but rather about my experiences and how they can help you. I want to share with you all the tools and secrets I've discovered, the lessons I've learned and the secrets I've uncovered through extensive research. I will also share enlightening insights drawn from people I have personally learned from.

I have taken what I have learned and written it down here so that you can get the most out of it. Almost everything I know about people is from observation, intuition, experience, and study. I am very empathetic and love to learn about different people and the qualities that make them special, and so I'll be sharing with you the best of what I have observed on developing a charismatic personality. It's fascinating!

My goal is to ignite something within you, to inspire you to become the best you can possibly be. However, I only wish you to use what you learn from me to help others—never to manipulate or take advantage. Taking advantage of others is incredibly bad karma, and it *will* come back to bite you.

Nothing has hurt my loving soul and gentle heart more than living among people who do not have the same ethics as me or who don't understand them. You cannot let negative situations and negative people take over and ruin your life. My life has not always been tranquil, and because of this, I constantly practice non-attachment, patience and forgiveness. Do not mistake my kindness for weakness; I put a lot of effort into being kind.

We must all make right what we can and accept what we cannot change, and then learn from it. I try to turn my misfortunes into opportunities, into lessons learned. Without them, this book would not exist. Humility builds character, and character is something that no one can give you—you have to earn it yourself. I've earned mine!

Each individual on this Earth holds concealed charisma within that needs to be discovered and kept alive, nurtured with the warmth of positivity and care. We are all charismatic, but we must keep a step ahead and stay focused on our passions, on becoming better people at our core. You already possess the charisma factor, and when you realize it, your efforts to carry its magnetism forward will be worth appreciating and developing. The French call this quality *je ne sais quoi*, or "I know not what."

We all possess charisma, and we all possess the charisma *factor*. We need only discover it within ourselves and share that positivity with the world. Too often, we become a product of the material world around us and lose sight of the fact that we are first and foremost spiritual beings. You can take away the body, but the spirit lives on. It is immortal, intangible. And so is your charisma factor—an unseen but powerful force that can help you shape your life for the better.

You need only spark the fire and keep it lit.

Chapter 1

Charisma Is Inside You

We all know that person who can just walk into a room and effortlessly command everybody's attention. Were they just born with this special ability? Or could you feasibly do the same?

It turns out that, yes, you *can* actually develop this magical quality yourself.

Charisma is a presence, one which sets people apart from one another. Those who possess the radiant power to understand and follow their chosen roads can really live and die as owners of charismatic personalities and lead prosperous, authentic and fulfilling lives. Of course, once charisma helps you in the door, you'll still need to also acquire the skills needed to keep that door open—but that's getting ahead of myself.

Charisma is that special, compelling spark within you that makes you who you are, different from the rest, with an ability to excite yourself and others.

The charisma factor is an amalgamation of your inherent talent, the passion with which you were born and the natural forces that when aligned, ignite your energy potential and soul.

The most common mistake most people make is to look for their charisma in the outer world, ignoring the truth that what they are searching for lies within. The yearning to develop charisma and grab hold of it leads one on a journey to find the supreme power that rests inside each of us. The ability to develop this captivating quality is something you already possess; you just need the tools necessary to mine it, nurture it and unleash it.

I have seen the power of charisma up close and personal. As an actress, I have many friends in Hollywood and have been introduced to many famous people from other areas and professions. Just as importantly, as an actress I have learned how to *portray* charisma and the power it both inspires and confers. In short, I am not only fascinated by this oft-misunderstood power but I have also felt it resonate through my psyche and my soul. It has captured my attention in a way nothing else has; I have felt its power and I have long desired to understand it from as many different perspectives as possible.

And not *just* understand it: my reason for writing this book was to help others understand what charisma really is…and one other mind-blowing concept: learning how you can develop your own charisma.

I have discovered that charisma is not only for leaders and celebrities, but is something that can be developed by anyone who has the interest, drive and the tools needed to make it happen. My passion about charisma has led me to research its role in many different spheres: history, artistic expression, psychology, and so on. I was surprised to learn that there was already a sizeable body of scientific literature about the topic.

These journeys into different fields allowed me to develop a clearer picture of what charisma is, and more importantly, how it can be developed. I learned a lot from my studies, and I want to pass on to you the fundamental truths that I have discovered on our shared journey towards ultimate empowerment.

I was in a meeting recently, expressing my views on the issue being discussed, and after I finished saying my piece, a colleague turned to me and said something I felt was very important: "Wow, Leesa!" she said, "You're on fire!"

On fire? Yes, absolutely! I felt so connected, so integrated in my heart, mind and soul. It was like all my circuits were working in harmony. I was fully aligned, and as soon as I was, the energy just flowed, effortlessly and relentlessly.

The meeting was for my Animal Ashram project, an endeavor which holds great meaning for me. I am passionate about the work we do there. It completely resonates with my purpose; I don't have to play a role when I'm there, I am just authentic—just me, passionate, completely engaged, and as a result, charismatic.

Charisma is a vivacity that no money can buy. It is an energy that can't be seen but can be felt, as can its real, tangible results. It fills us up with a positivity that cannot be shackled by negative energy. This is how it also encourages us to remain calm, composed, gracious, focused, and optimistic. Radiance dominates when we stay away from anger, evil thoughts, frustration, and jealousy.

The formula for developing this "charisma factor" is very simple. If you want to excel in anything, you need to have a passion for it. If you want to make your presence known in a particular sphere, it helps to have a natural talent for the thing you are pursuing. Once you know you're good at something, feel passionate about it, and are sure you would like to pursue it as your chosen path, all that is necessary is to hone your skills, perfect your craftsmanship.

People like President Donald Trump, John F. Kennedy Jr., Taylor Swift, Michael Jackson, and Princess Diana aren't the only ones who have this "Charisma Factor." *Everyone* is born with this inherent characteristic. What we need to do is to delve into ourselves to find our own distinctive quality, and we'll surely find it sooner or later if we look for it honestly within ourselves. No one can undertake this search for us. It is solely our own responsibility to find out more about this unique quality hidden within us.

Each of our own distinguishing charisma factor comprises a synergy of talent, personal magnetism, empathy and passion that connects us to our ultimate goals. It may take some time to find, so you'll need to be patient if you're serious about discovering yourself. You need to plan out time to devote to the search and keep yourself motivated until you find that special component. Just know that the closer you get to it, the more positive energy you will feel encompassing you.

Once you connect to your inner self, you will know who you are, which will give you a new sense of identity. This awareness will help put you on the right track to solve problems in your life that have bothered you for years, perhaps even all your life. When you no longer feel the urge to run away from your problems, when you no longer hide from yourself or from the world outside, you'll be giving yourself the courage to face all the odds of life. Solving difficult problems is what defines us. We can use our creativity and thinking power to resolve our troubles one after the other, depending on their intensity and proportion.

All of us have the capacity to do this; the difference is just that those who start the process early in their lives will be the first to achieve their goals. But whether you're just starting out in life or reinventing yourself, you can start right this moment to succeed in your own way. Connecting to your true self and understanding what you really desire to achieve are the first challenges. Relate to yourself from within to find the truth that lies buried deep inside you, as this process will pave the way for you to recognize your passion, that knack for a particular objective that you choose to pursue.

The positive magnetism in humanity is reflected through our different mediums of expression. Sometimes it comes directly from someone's alluring beauty, sometimes it's the magical vocal cords that enchant all who listen. Sometimes, the charisma factor reflects through someone's artistic character, and sometimes it's just their smile that's charismatic enough to heal wounded hearts. The gleam of existence shines through each of these creations and flourishes, which is what allows it to reach its highest level and to triumph over all obstacles. This illuminating quality is inside every individual and nurturing it forever with goodness and strength will make it grow and glow.

The desire to discover charisma urges us to seek the most charismatic and creative people, who spread their wisdom generously to others. Have you ever noticed someone whose body echoed irresistible charm? Have you heard such a powerful voice that it swung like a shrill sword, piercing the air around you and entering your earlobes to touch the frailest slice of your soul? Has the magnetism of someone's charismatic presence influenced a desire in you to become more like that person? Moreover, have you found yourself on a constant hunt for the way out of the darkness in which you're living to reach the level of prosperity and purpose someone enjoys by being charismatic?

The yearning to develop the power of charisma is too powerful to be escaped—an irresistible desire that draws us towards the charismatic people in our lives like bees to honey. But the gleaming sunshine of positivity and inspiration that holds us so enthralled is no mere coincidence; it is a result of self-awareness, enduring drive and boundless passion. Charisma is both source and symptom of success, and the essence of this supreme power can only be found by searching within your soul.

Chapter 2

Are You Born with Charisma?

The question of whether charisma is an inborn trait or something that can be acquired has been long debated. It was once thought that charisma was a quality that was present only in people with blue blood, like royalty; others believed that only religious leaders and celebrities possessed it, something regarded as a divine gift not given to everybody. But this outlook, besides ignoring the facts of the matter, strikes me as defeatist. There is much that speaks to the contrary of this school of thought, and it's my opinion that while some people do seem to have a knack for influencing others, *charisma can be consciously enhanced.*

Luminaries such as Abraham Lincoln, John F. Kennedy, Gandhi, and Martin Luther King, Jr. worked hard on their charisma to achieve their goals. These are people who rose to the challenge and never let themselves stay down. Some might call this 'the theory of attribution at work.' This theory states that your perception of the world can have influence on others.

Gandhi, for instance, rose from a very humble background to teach the world a lesson. Gandhi's magnetic charisma developed because he saw the truth and allowed it to dominate his personality. He knew that he could not achieve his goals without the steely determination to commit to achieving what he set out to do. He never turned his back on his sense of self or his origins while spreading his philosophy to others, and it was that quiet confidence he maintained in observing the truth around him that created his charisma—his aura of influence—that no one could touch or quite put their finger on. They saw that he spoke the truth but were at a loss for how to achieve the same thing.

In discussing these eminent personalities, it becomes obvious that they saw the world differently than those around them; in some cases, they were way ahead of their times. But they slowly encouraged the masses to believe in what they did, and because of their insightfulness, they made an impact on others and had a profound effect on the situations in which they found themselves.

HOW CAN YOU ACQUIRE CHARISMA?

If charisma is not inborn, then how can it be cultivated? Is charisma something that can be practiced? Are there steps to take or a school to attend that can teach you how to be charismatic? While I know of no single institution that offers a degree in charisma, the answer is yes: it *can* be learned and, of course, practiced. All you need is the true grit to learn it by yourself, practicing over and over until it becomes a part of your daily life. You must consciously get into the habit of being charismatic and charming. More details about how to become charismatic are included in the workbook at the back of the book, but for now, consider these ideas for learning the art of charisma:

Be knowledgeable. Martin Luther King, Jr. was valedictorian of his class before he became the most visible figure in the Civil Rights movement. Knowledge can always help you become enlightened and will never deceive you. It can also assist you in connecting with your inner peace and self. Admittedly, the search for knowledge will take time, but can facilitate the attainment of charisma.

Be open to change. Nature is dynamic, and if there's one thing that never stops in this world, it's change. Charismatic people are generally open to change and can adapt themselves well. In fact, they often lend a hand to others, helping them to adjust. Therefore, if you want to learn the art of charisma, you need to embrace the transformations around you and work hard to bring some about within yourself.

Be honest. Be true to yourself and to others. Truth can bring a glow to your system, both internally and externally. There's no reason to pretend while trying to please others. Honesty, indeed, is the best policy. There's no point in running away from the truth, and you can resolve the biggest mysteries in the world by remaining honest with yourself. Your honesty makes you authentic, and it will make you appear pure in the eyes of your audience.

Listen to others. Most of us either try to dominate others or drive them away by saying what they don't want to hear. We often become too bored or impatient to really listen to others.

It isn't easy to find true listeners in this world, but when you come across them, you know they'll at least let you have your say. Going forward, you know whom to go to when you're feeling low or depressed. That's what the magic of listening is all about. Learn to be a patient listener; only then will you be able to provide people with solutions to their problems. That will certainly make you different from the rest.

Keep a warm and pleasant smile. Charismatic personalities wear warm smiles wherever they go, spreading positive energy to everyone they encounter. A genuine, smiling face always looks good, makes people feel better around you, and adds charm to your personality.

Offer a helping hand. Offering sincere assistance can make you look more charismatic in the eyes of others. What matters here is making the offer; whether someone accepts it isn't the important part. Your offer shows that you're attempting to make a difference. Remember, not everyone may want to accept your energy. It's up to you to make peace with that.

Appreciate others. Everyone wants to hear a word of appreciation now and then. It lets them know that someone is taking notice of them and what they do. For this reason, complimenting others is one of the best ways to connect with them; your positive words contribute to getting to know them.

These are just a few things you can focus on to build your charisma. Remember to always focus on your strengths and let them do the talking. That way, you'll create a ring of positivity around you that will help channel your energy in the right direction.

IS CHARISMA GENETIC?

There may be some genetic factors related to charisma. Your looks, intelligence, and health are traits that can be passed down through generations, and have positive correlation with charismatic personalities. But I'm sure we can all think of examples of charismatic people who weren't blessed with perfect looks, or who had physical disabilities. I strongly believe we are all born with a spark of charisma; we need only find it within ourselves and slowly and steadily reveal it to the world.

SOCIETY AS A CHARISMA BUILDER

Sociologically speaking, your family, peers, government, and religion are all facets of life which help shape your inner charisma. These social ties keep you going and protect you from negative forces in a host of different ways. You idealize your parents, appreciate your friends and colleagues, receive civic rights from the government, and learn right from wrong through your religion. None of these social institutions *force* you to follow the norms that have existed for centuries, but all of them hold one thing in common: they can guide you towards candor, self-actualization and integrity. Your family teaches you to be dedicated; your peers coach you about loyalty; your religion trains you in devotion; and your government instructs you on personal and collective responsibility. This is how we learn about life and gather up the building blocks for our own charismatic personalities.

My grandfather on my mother's side handled my parents' divorce. He was a very tough attorney who'd never lost a case and he was tough with my father. It happened when I was six; I was not allowed to see my father again until my eighteenth birthday. By then, I felt abandoned by my father. I prayed nightly to see him again; missing him was agony. I thought I would give anything for one more day with him.

When he died of a heart attack over decade ago, my sister and I were the ones who cleared out his drawers. There, we found numerous returned letters asking to visit us, along with paintings, drawings, and mementos from our early childhood, and all the letters he saved that we had written him.

I never knew who my biological father was, and still don't. I used to look at the kids in school and wonder if there was some way we could be related. My grandfather was like a father to me, too, and I loved him dearly. But he died of cancer when I was sixteen. I had an especially hard time mourning his passing, which is what led to my beginning to meditate and read up on all things related to spirituality.

I have obviously had issues and have done continual, deep soul searching throughout my life. I battle the fear of abandonment and have felt distressingly crushed by my emotions at times. I don't find it easy to share my problems with others, so I really have had to draw on and develop my inner charisma factor to help me persevere and clear my mind's fog. I choose to see the positive in everything around me and refuse to become bitter. It is true what people say: excruciating times build character.

How can you practice charisma and build character on your own? Some people are lucky enough to have mentors, while others teach themselves. I have done and continue to do both. You're free to choose whatever strategy seems appropriate for you. I find that self-discovery is the best way to master just about anything relating to consciousness, including charisma. It's the best way I've found to learn more, question more, and seek more answers.

That being said, while coaches can help you understand ideas, they shouldn't spoon-feed the answers to you. You must have the hunger to master the trait of charisma, and ideally, you'll satisfy it by feeding yourself with knowledge. That is why the choice of a charisma teacher is so important. Your progress will accelerate—exponentially so—with a teacher to guide you, so long as they are the right teacher for you.

Chapter 3

Can Charisma Be Refined?

You will be glad to know that charisma can be consciously learned and enhanced and brought out, whether by a teacher, a healer, or through conscious self-exploration. I consider myself an eternal student and am constantly seeking knowledge from various "teachers". The only thing that a teacher needs to be sure of is that their student wants to learn and can be trained to bring out their charismatic personality.

As for what the student requires, they must of course to be focused. Focus is the most significant element that you, as a student of the art of charisma, will need. Your concentration and will to learn can do wonders.

As a student, you will also need to be patient. You must know that things will not happen right away; it will take time to show results when you learn any art, but all of us are born with charisma, though only a few will find it in themselves.

You will also benefit from a clarity of purpose. Often you may find yourself wondering during the process: why do you want to become charismatic in the first place? Maybe you wish to transcend your long-time personal limitations, but the best answer I've found is to be able to contribute to society in a meaningful way. Many people are highly qualified, educated, and well-trained...but despite this, they still feel that they inherently lack something.

Their work is skillful, meticulous; they are hardworking and goal-oriented, but still they are not well-recognized or appreciated. Perhaps they've gotten passed over for promotions, maybe they cannot seem to hold people's attention when they speak, or they just never seem to land the type of role they're dying to play.

They lack the consideration they deserve with respect to their work. Instead, the recognition they deserve has been given to someone else—who may be less educated or experienced.

What these people lack isn't luck or talent—it's charisma.

Many people associate charisma only with having a great personality, thinking people with charisma are charming, attractive, excellent speakers with great fan followings and influence on others. On the contrary—charismatic people need not be famous, attractive, or rich. Charisma is something that is not defined by or limited to just celebrities and elites. A schoolteacher can be charismatic, if their students admire them and want to follow along in the lesson. In the workplace, a colleague in a lower position can be more popular and admired than someone in a higher position, and so on.

This is because *true* charisma is actually about projecting your best self with self-respect and dignity. This projection is an active skill, not a passive trait; this is why charisma can be present one moment and absent the very next. The magic appears only when one wants to exhibit it. One can simply go unnoticed if he or she does not want attention just by changing their gestures or body language. It is a person's choice what they want to project.

This is why research has shown that charisma is a set of behaviors, rather than an inherent personal quality. In other words, charisma can be learned and acquired like any other social skill. Sometimes, people won't even notice that they are learning to be more charismatic. They try new behaviors, see better results, and gradually these more effective behaviors become instinctive. When we see a charismatic personality, we rarely appreciate that we're seeing a finished product, something that has been fought for and labored over. We don't see them struggling along the way. One thing is always certain, though: as a result of this behind the scenes struggle, those who now shine do so by having learned to connect with their charismatic selves.

Great people learn to develop charismatic personalities and grow them over time. To this end, some people will hire coaches or mentors to help them do this; others learn on their own. You are free to choose which way you want to go but no matter how many mentors you work with, it will still be up to you to find *your* charisma and connect to *your* inner self.

Richard Wiseman, a British professor of psychology, has extensively researched charisma. His conclusion is that charismatic people influence others positively. His study included more than 200 people taking part in a national competition called FameLab. Its goal: to find the new "faces of science." In FameLab, contestants would have 3 minutes to win over their audience and judges with a scientific talk using charisma, clarity and content. He noticed that his subjects either copied the physical styles or words of their idols. This influence is not superficial; by imitating style or words, people connect to their own charisma and inner selves, reflecting what they like. This means the positive aspects of the people they like begin to influence them positively, slowly integrating more of that external positive into their own internal lives.

Professor Wiseman further states that learning to be charismatic means acquiring certain skills. Once you acquire these skills, though, you will still need to continue to practice them. (See the charisma workbook on page 111 to get yourself started.) You need to be present in the moment to get acclamation from others. You need to listen to people, use good body language, and speak clearly. You should be self-motivated, confident, and strong-willed to accomplish your task.

People will remember the charismatic people they've met, long after they are gone from the world. Make a choice about the impression you want to leave behind: Would you imprint it with your thoughts, like a famous writer or philosopher? Would you like to be known for your style and grace, as a fashion icon or taste maker? Would you leave behind a legacy of inspiring speeches, or courageous acts?

If you really want to be charismatic, then you need to identify the traits in charismatic people you'd like to emulate. You need to be focused on your mission and keep learning in the process. Yes, charisma can be learned and developed. Constantly following your mind and heart and keeping an eye on what you want to achieve and who you ultimately want to become is what will help you acquire charisma.

The desire to discover charisma is strongest when you observe charismatic people around you. When you see them spreading their magic, when you hear their irresistible, charming words, and when their magnetism attracts everyone around them, you notice their charisma. The sheer pleasure of being in someone charismatic's presence makes you want to be like that person. You are mesmerized by the thought of the prosperity they enjoy by being charismatic and having influence over people.

Believe that that same charisma is somewhere in you; it is just configured differently in each of us. You may have beauty, luck, reputation, and charm, yet still lack the magnetic attraction of charisma. You might wonder why you seem to have everything, but are not more admired than others. You may have all these things, but you might need some tips from others to make yourself more charismatic. You just have to decide what kind of change you want in yourself and prepare to work for it.

Charisma also differs with personality type, and the way people present it is also very different. No two human beings are alike, and neither are charismatic personalities. For instance, try to compare Presidents Trump, Clinton, and Kennedy. They are all charismatic, but each in his own unique way. We can develop charisma by studying the behavior of charismatic personalities, while keeping in mind that these are individuals, not cookie-cutter personalities.

By the time you are done reading this book, I want you to have learned to believe in the charisma factor within you. I know you are a unique, individual soul, present on this earth for some specific purpose. There is no formula or magic pill that can ignite charisma in you. There is no set of standards or any code of conduct to follow that will kindle it. It is a slow and steady process of self-discovery which enlightens one's very own purpose for being here. For true charisma to blossom, one has to discover one's purpose and accomplish it.

I like to say, whether you think you can or cannot be charismatic, either way…you are right.

Always remember: *you possess charisma.* It just requires the right ignition, a small spark. No matter how much you want to be charismatic, if you cannot discover the key to this ignition within you, you will just end up admiring others.

Know yourself and try to wake yourself so that you can meet your best self. Learn from everything you can; get inspired by whomever you can, but understand that the bottom line is to know yourself and learn. You can develop and create charisma. It is not rare or impossible; the only thing required to find yours is attention to your capabilities.

As a result of your new-found charisma, you may find new meaning in life, and you may actually start making a difference in the lives of others. Helping others offers the kind of contentment that can bring you true inner peace. There is nothing better than this feeling.

One of my favorite quotes is from Swami Vivekananada, and sums this up nicely: "Condemn none: if you can stretch out a helping hand, do so. If you cannot, fold your hands, bless your brothers, and let them go their own way."

The following are a few things that you can do along this journey towards a whole new realization of yourself. (For more specific guidance, refer to the workbooks on page 111.)

Use your power. Use power in different ways according to your objective, but remember that power used in the noblest ways brings the best results. Power is implemented and expressed through our language and actions without us even realizing it, but others who judge us will notice these actions.

The best thing to do is to train yourself to be more confident. Confidence helps you face judgment with courage and confers the power to deal with all kinds of different people.

Confidence also helps you accomplish things you've always wanted. By developing your willpower to achieve the impossible, you will come to believe that *nothing* is impossible. You will try new things and find success again and again. Where you don't immediately succeed, you still won't give up. Willpower becomes a driving force; you will keep trying the things you fail at, only to succeed at them later through hard work.

The power of intention becomes an important motive force in shaping your charisma. It is your life's purpose that matters. So, if you keep a positive goal in your mind, if you can *see* it happen, things will go in your favor. Such is the power of belief in yourself when paired with hard work.

Show warmth. The least we can do for others is to show warmth. Your goodwill reflects in your actions. Often, people will not understand your behavior, or may find it difficult to get a read on your personality. But when you display your friendly nature, the barrier between you and the rest of the world breaks down. Your warm and sweet smile can make all the difference in the world. After all, it is very hard to find people without a smile of kindness.

Be mindful of your behavior. Many believe that you can change your behavior, but not your personality. Working on behavior is a key element while learning to develop your charismatic self. This means your body language must be equally convincing when you try to project your hospitable self. Half the battle will be won if you learn how to do this correctly. Everyone has their share of problems in their lives. If someone shows a little love and care, people will be captivated. There is no harm in talking to people nicely, and once you realize this, you will help your charisma to come out in the open.

Be present. To be present, gather your thoughts and concentrate on the present moment. You need to be present in the *present* moment, which means you cannot allow your mind to drift away at all. People will believe in you only if you believe in yourself; in the same way, being present always and staying focused on the situation at hand will make others more inclined to trust you.

One way to increase your power of concentration is to meditate. This really is the best tool that you can use for giving yourself that extra boost in focus. Meditation helps you connect to the real you. It is a means by which many millions of people throughout history have found the true happiness hidden inside themselves. You may not know what exactly brings you joy now, but by meditating, you will come to know for sure. The purpose of your being here will become very clear, which will give you a reason to be content.

Charisma can be taught only to those who are willing to learn. The student must motivate themselves to learn; however, they must also have endurance—the fortitude to carve their way toward the realization of their true potential.

Next, let's examine some of the lessons new students of charisma will be expected to learn—and master—on their road to becoming truly charismatic. And so we must ask, what is it that makes a person appear charismatic to others?

Chapter 4

What Makes a Person Charismatic?

"If you want to be happy, practice compassion. If you want others to be happy, practice compassion."

—Buddha

I have always been an observer and people watcher; I love to study what makes people unique. And since I am so intrigued with charisma, I'm always looking for the nuances of what gives a person that sense of charismatic magnetism.

From my own observations, I have found there are many facets to charisma and many ways of being charismatic, but they always return to that most important principle: to always be true to your own unique self. The following are a few key concepts designed to help you express your unique self, while also provoking thought as to how you can improve on your best qualities.

Always be authentic. Don't try fake charm to impress others or even yourself. Remember, no one was born yesterday and there's nothing charismatic about a phony. Charisma is a force, one that you cannot hide or fake; it's a quality that radiates from inside.

Remain determined. Everyone has heard the story of the high-paid actor or actress in Hollywood who was once a struggling waiter or waitress. This is true—many of the well-known celebrities you see in the movies today had to put in a *lot* of hard work before their careers took off. There were times when they had to roll up their sleeves and earn a living in different, far less glamorous occupations.

The truth of the "overnight success" is that it can take years to achieve, and the same is true for charisma. I was an actress in Hollywood in the late eighties through the mid-nineties and have remained friends with several renowned actors and actresses during their highs and lows. The truth is that reality does bite us all at one time or another.

So, if you really want to know what brings out the charisma in a person, the answer is: sheer determination. If you have strong determination to accomplish your goals, nothing will stand in your way. You will be able to pass every hurdle in your path to achieve your dream.

Be open to change. Although not everyone is open to change, those who adapt according to the demands of the times come the closest to being charismatic. This is probably why there are very few truly successful people: they lead from the front, and we follow. Being adaptable is a hugely important ingredient, and changing your attitude to reflect this can make a tremendous difference.

Try it today. There's no time like the present. You might start by dressing in a way that makes you feel more confident or attractive. You could even consult a stylist. The point is to try something new that might work for you. At worst, come tomorrow you'll be able to say you tried, whether the new way works for you or not. If you want different results, you must do something different. (Refer to the first section of the workbook on behavior change for tips on how to get started.)

Keep your thoughts pure and your body clean. Always keep your thoughts clean and pure by thinking constructively. Think well of others and concentrate on the positives. I constantly say to myself, "Love and light" and, "Breathe in peace, breathe out love". Clean thoughts can free the mind to think for the good of all. Remember that we create our world through our thoughts.

Maintaining good hygiene is also part of bringing out your best charismatic self. Be sure to bathe every day. Water can cleanse your body of negative energies; it *is* a universal solvent, after all. Cleansing has a deeper meaning than you might think: it keeps you fresh and protected. I generally take a long bath in the morning and often another in the evening because it helps me relax and focus on what is important to me. I see it as a sort of meditation.

Finally, be sure to tend to your energy—your aura—which should be kept clean for best results. Keeping a positive approach toward life can help you do this. Learning and reading about charismatic personalities or the top leaders of the world can also serve as inspiration. This will unquestionably keep your aura clean in the best possible ways.

Develop taste. You need to develop your intelligence and perception if you aim to excel in life. Read good literature, learn about beautiful art, stay up-to-date on current affairs, and wear neat and well-tailored clothes. There is a saying in Sanskrit: "a king's respect is limited to his kingdom, but a learned man is respected everywhere." Keep that in mind, and you'll be motivated to keep learning to become cultured and well-read.

Be approachable. Making yourself more approachable doesn't mean that you should crack cheap jokes or get overly friendly with everyone. This type of behavior can cause others discomfort. A charismatic personality is one who knows how to strike the balance between being friendly and being overly friendly. They never overdo anything and inherently know when to talk and when to stop. This is most certainly an art form, one that will come to you with time and practice. For a starter, try maintaining a warm, genuine smile on your face. A smile inclines people to connect with you. When your smile is genuine, you'll get attention in a crowd from the warmth you exude.

Stay humble. Always make it a point to control your emotions and be very careful with the way you react to things. A charismatic person's behavior is not dictatorial or autocratic, so avoid dominating others or showing self-importance. Adolf Hitler is the classic example of a man who made this mistake. He used his charisma in an enormously damaging way. A brilliant orator, he not only managed to charm the whole of Germany, but at one point almost the entire world. If he could have used his charisma for good, the history of the world would have been totally different.

Listen to others. When listening to other people, do so with your full attention. Everyone likes to be listened to, and in this busy world, great listeners are hard to come by. True listening could probably solve half the problems of the world. It's because so many of us are too busy talking about ourselves that we find few truly attentive listeners. It was said that former president Bill Clinton was a great listener, and this contributed to his charismatic influence and overwhelming popularity.

Speak well. Talking about positive things and using the right body language allows you to effectively communicate your thoughts and ideas to others, inspiring them to do the same. No one likes a show-off, so know your limits and learn the correct method of speaking well. But if you are well-read, communication will come more naturally to you, and you'll know more about a variety of topics. Be sensible and speak honorably to people of all ages and from all backgrounds.

Which isn't to say speaking well extends only to professional or academic discussions. At times, an optimistic word of encouragement offered to another person is all someone may be looking for. Your words may have the power to change a life forever by serving as a catalyst for change. I try to have a positive impact on the lives of others and always look for the good in people, rather than be critical.

Improve eye contact. Start looking those you meet in the eye straight away. Make sure that your gaze isn't too long—that can scare or intimidate people—but don't make it too short either; that may seem abrupt. Just look into people's eyes until you get a good idea of their eye color; that's a helpful gauge.

Practice this with your family and friends if you're uncertain; after all, practice makes perfect.

Respect people's personal space. Develop your ability to make people comfortable so they feel secure in your presence. Anthropologist Edward Hall believed that humans consider their personal space threatened the moment we hear someone speaking about us, looking us in the eye, physically touching us (with a pat or a rub), standing right in front of us, or even raising their voice at us.

However, some of these things can be done in a positive way, and many charismatic people have the ability to channel these actions into something mesmerizing, rather than threatening. For example, when calling someone by name or patting someone on the shoulder, make it a point to stand at an angle to them. This will lessen the intimidating effect.

Learn the art of being present. Think of how many times your mind has drifted away while you were talking to somebody. This is sometimes called a pretend gaze, because while you may be in the same room with them, you're really miles away, thinking about paying your bills or your last vacation or just noticing items in the room—or even thinking about the next person you want to talk to. This is something great listeners like Oprah Winfrey and President Donald Trump, for instance, would never do. They ensure that when they're listening to you, they're attentive, making you feel there's no one else in the world they'd rather be listening to at that moment.

Show compassion. Another way of making your presence felt and memorable is by showing compassion—something that can't be faked. I'm a trained actress and understand very well the importance of empathy; however, true empathy is something that doesn't come naturally to everyone. The simplest way to begin developing a compassionate attitude is to compliment others and refrain from judging them. The moment you start noticing the good in others, they'll do the same for you. If you talk to someone nicely, chances are that person will reciprocate.

These are just a few of the secret weapons you can use to project your charisma. A blend of all these factors will aid in developing this trait and help you achieve your goals. If you want to appeal to people, then first you need to know how to be a "people person" and learn to break the ice between you and others in small, charismatic ways.

Chapter 5

Charismatic Personalities

The magnetism of charismatic people goes very deep. It has often been said that they can light up any room that they have entered without even speaking. They have a power by which they radiate positive energy, which is what captures everyone's attention. Each of us has certainly come across such personalities in our own lives.

According to many ancient philosophies, the human body is the quintessence of five major elements: earth, water, spirit, fire, and air. These components together construct human existence, deciding the functions and nature of our body. Hence, these elements play prominent roles in discovering our own unique charisma. Those who can unlock the secrets of these elements, and explore their inner charisma factor can, quite simply, accomplish their innermost desires of being charismatic forever.

Many famous charismatic personalities across the globe have understood this fact, in some way or another, and have either worked hard to develop the charisma factor in themselves or worked adequately to retain the talent they were born with. It's said that charisma is rare; however, I believe it's simply rarely discovered.

Do you really think you're different from someone you view as charismatic?

How is it possible this person was endowed with enchanting qualities you don't have a chance of developing? We are all born with the same basic elements. Isn't there a similar process by which both your hearts pump blood through your bodies? Don't you both possess a number of emotions, likes and dislikes, have important things to say, and the desire for the warmth of love and affection? Of course you do!

Reality television personality Lisa Gastineau feels that "a woman with charisma has the special "it" factor that attracts others into her mind and shows how she ticks. This virtue can easily out-shadow others with more social status, beauty, fame and wealth."

If things are similar in every human being, why are only a few of us getting noticed? Primarily, the answer is that others have already discovered the key to charisma within themselves and you haven't. That's the basic difference that sets you apart from those special and gifted people.

To remove the thin line of difference between you and them, all you need to do is remember that your life has a mission and that whatever that mission may be, it can't be completed without exploring the charismatic power you hold inside. Once you begin to discover the guiding light that lies within you, all you need to do is to keep your enthusiasm level high and keep yourself motivated. This will help you to continue without halting until you have achieved success.

There have been countless magnetic people throughout the past centuries, and there will be more to come. Across the globe, luminaries and charismatic personalities have been successful in making their names recognized and their popularity spread. The list can go on indefinitely.

In the following chapters I discuss and analyze some of my favorite personalities and the qualities they possess that I have deemed their "charisma factors." Let's begin with one of my personal favorites, Princess Diana.

PRINCESS DIANA

This beautiful princess, born in 1961, had it all in the beginning: she had a fairy-tale wedding, and her Prince Charming was a real prince. As time passed, she realized that her fairy tale was coming to an end on a bitter note. Once it did, she paid a heavy price. Her tragic demise in 1997 made even people who didn't know her mourn her passing. That was her charisma, yet all she wanted was to be remembered as someone who cared for the needy. Yes, she did succeed in her mission, and to this day, she is remembered as a charismatic personality.

Initially dubbed "Shy Di," during her reign, she made it her mission to turn that image around and eventually became a global icon. Her presence grew to become very powerful, combined with her beauty, and ended up producing something explosive. She became the quintessential symbol of the twentieth-century woman who had modern values with a humanitarian touch.

Diana, Princess of Wales, had empathy for people, which is something one needs to immediately connect to the crowd.

In my opinion, that was the quality she possessed that enabled her to be so successfully involved in social work. There is no need to explain that her presence at charity events promoted awareness as well as fetched monetary gains that were used to help others.

She had charm, yet she was vulnerable; she had the warmth and vivacity to help others. She was passionate about her humanitarian activities and eradicating AIDS, which was a very pressing concern at the time, was at the top of her agenda. Along with this cause, she took up another mission: to eliminate landmines, as she had seen their consequences. She also had a soft spot concerning diseases that had rendered people "untouchable" in the past, including leprosy. She lent her time to all kinds of issues that had been brushed under the carpet for centuries, which is why she is often referred to as "the people's princess." Her charismatic personality was more than enough to influence people and get them to believe in her causes.

Her leadership skills were excellent, proving she was a princess who could relate to the general population. She changed the way people looked at the monarchy.

Before her death, it seemed as if she had found a profound reason to live and share her wisdom and warmth. She was on a mission that she didn't want to let go of and became more absorbed in it as time passed. She had a unique way of comforting the people around her, which is why they accepted her as "the people's princess" in no time at all. Her compassion was very authentic, which is why people had faith in her.

Princess Diana had an ever-growing fan base all across the world. She had sympathy on her side because her personal life was going in the wrong direction People empathized with her because of her bitter divorce, and the reasons for it were quite evident to the whole world.

After her separation from the prince, some people started to blame her for the mishap. The media wouldn't allow her to live in peace, but she used this attention to deflect the focus from her personal life toward her charitable interests. She soon regained popularity and even helped a few journalists to write about her life. All this kept adding to her support, until one night when she went into that fatal Paris tunnel and died under very questionable circumstances.

Her charisma was relative: she could relate to people, and they could relate to her. She was supported by the world, and she returned the favor in all possible ways. She could bond with people very quickly because she had found her happiness in them, free of affectation and any kind of showing off. She lived an open life and never tried to hide herself, which is another reason why people liked her. They could see through to her, which added to her popularity.

I believe Princess Diana was the epitome of feminine beauty with a dash of power. She set an example for many. She was the woman who took on a traditionalist Britain, forcing it to change with her modern values.

If we learn nothing else from her, it should be that you always have a chance to turn things around; life gives us second chances. She took her second chance and converted her life into something she was zealous about. She dedicated her life to the people, and they made her their own princess. She believed that everyone should be valued and showed how that could really be done, holding the hands of people stricken with AIDS at a time when many believed the disease could be spread through casual contact.

Her charisma was an amalgamation of beauty, charm, honesty, and care. This explains why 2.5 billion people all over the world viewed her funeral on television. Indeed, to this day, she remains special royalty for the people.

We can all learn from the example Princess Diana set with the way she lived her life. Look deep within your soul and your mind and find what is important to you. Stand up for your convictions. Be honest, tenacious, and authentic. Choose to help others or speak up for those who can't speak for themselves when you are fortunate enough to have the opportunity to do so.

Let's continue our exploration of these fascinating personalities and discover what made them so uniquely charismatic in the next chapter.

CHRIS DEROSE

Chris DeRose, born June 28, 1948, in Brooklyn, New York, is the founder and president of the national animal rights nonprofit Last Chance for Animals and is one of the most charismatic people I know. I met him in Los Angeles when I was nineteen and have always felt inspired by him.

At age five, Chris went into an orphanage in New Jersey, and later made his home there and became an investigator and police officer. He gave up a very lucrative acting career in Los Angeles to stand up for his convictions and fight for animals, who are also charismatic creatures. He exudes charisma and uses it to benefit others, not to feed his ego, or use others, or profit financially.

Chris has used his passion and charismatic personality to become an international leader in the animal rights movement and is focused on investigating, exposing, and ending animal exploitation. He has been arrested twelve times and jailed four times for opposing animal cruelty. He is the author of In Your Face: From Actor to Animal Activist and was also a special correspondent for television's Hard Copy.

Chris participated in a break-in at the UCLA Brain Research Institute in 1988, which was aired on CNN. It was responsible for shedding light on the vivisection that goes on behind the locked doors of research facilities.

He has put his life on the line for his beliefs, has been shot at and jailed for standing up for his personal convictions. He was a true pioneer in the animal rights movement in the early eighties and founded Last Chance for Animals in 1984. He has established himself as a leader in the animal rights movement and received the 1997 Peace Abbey Courage of Conscience Award.

Part of Chris's charisma factor is that he uses his passion, talent, and drive to make a positive difference in the lives of countless animals as well as people. Directing your life toward helping others who aren't fortunate enough to have a voice leads to more personal fulfillment, as well as extending your charismatic influence into the world.

ABRAHAM LINCOLN

"I destroy my enemies when I make them my friends" is an oft-quoted comment made by the sixteenth president of the United States. Abraham Lincoln, who was born in 1809 and died by assassination in 1865, was truly a charismatic man, although he always believed himself to be as ordinary as any other individual on earth, thus showing humility which is so much art of charisma.

He had the talent for recognizing his duties and mustering the strength to accomplish them. He was the kind of leader that everyone aspires to be, so special a man that people have been reading books about him for more than a century. People who want to learn the major skills of leadership study Lincoln's ideas and their implementation. His magnetism was something he was born with, but he carried it forward well because of his good deeds. His gift of grace made him one of the most celebrated American presidents.

Lincoln's words were magical, carrying such an appeal that they could entrap anyone, convincing them effectively. He would always say, "Whatever you are, be a good one," which explains that his charisma rested in his goodness. Despite being an average-looking man, he had the power to allure people with his presence, which is one of the reasons he still has a huge following, especially in politics.

Those who have the misconception that only attractive and good-looking people can be charismatic need only look at this man for their answer. He had neither conventional, gorgeous looks nor an attractive smile, yet the goodness within him made his charisma factor shine through. And though he is no longer physically present on this earth, his timeless charisma and ability to change the world for good is still alive well into the twenty-first century.

Lincoln always believed in one religion—humanity—but he had such a strong charisma factor that it glorified his persona. His saying, "When I do well, I feel good; when I do bad, I feel bad. That's my religion," is a rebuttal to those who are desperate to prove that charisma belongs only to a particular faith.

Learn to implement your ideas, be humble, develop empathy for others, speak well, and mean well. By doing so, you can make a big difference in your life as well as in the lives of others.

MALALA YOUSAFZAI

Malala Yousafzai, born July 12, 1997, is a young woman who burst onto the international stage in October of 2012 after coming face-to-face at the age of fifteen with an adversary that she had never imagined. Malala became the target of a Taliban assassin's bullet to the head because of a blog she had penned and interviews she had given to try to document and expose the challenges of young women who wanted to attend school in the Swat Valley of Pakistan. When she recovered from this horrific act, she took off afresh, finding all sorts of opportunities to bring light to these struggles. She seized the day. There was nothing to stop her at that point.

It was through adversity that she truly found her calling in life, and in the span of little more than a year, she found herself nominated for a Nobel Peace Prize that acknowledged her remarkable abilities to tell her story and shed light on the plights of young women in Taliban- controlled areas of Pakistan and elsewhere who struggle to be able to simply attend school.

A fund was set up in Malala's name to promote education for young people everywhere. A UN petition was created using the slogan "I am Malala" urging that all children in the world be freely allowed to attend school by 2015. She signed a $3 million book deal for her story. Malala even wound up on the front cover of Time magazine in 2013 as one of the 100 most influential people in the world.

You may ask how a petite, fifteen-year-old girl can achieve so much in so little time. It was obvious that for a while she even doubted how she could do it herself. She was quoted as saying, "Once I had asked God for one or two extra inches in height, but instead he made me as tall as the sky, so high that I could not measure myself." It is obvious that by then, Malala had found her own charisma factor—that thing that lay inside her that was about to light up the world!

It took an assassin's bullet to make Malala realize that she had all the strength she needed laying right inside of her—and it is highly unlikely this young girl's star will ever fade.

DONALD J. TRUMP

Larger-than-life personality Donald J. Trump was born on June 14, 1946 in Queens, NY, the fourth out of five children to Mary MacLeod and Frederick Christ Trump.

He attended the New York Military Academy from 1959–1964 and received a bachelor's degree in economics from the University of Pennsylvania's Wharton School of Finance and Commerce in 1968, shortly before taking up the reins of his family's real estate business in 1971.

Renaming the firm The Trump Organization, he expanded the business into Manhattan and Brooklyn, building hotels, skyscrapers, golf courses and casinos not only in New York but across the world. And, owing to his charismatic personality, glamour, and reputation as a developer, he was able to license his name to several developments in addition to his own.

Former President Trump has managed to combine his education with his charismatic appeal to create a very rare combination which in turn has enabled him to realize huge aspirations as well as pushing himself to the limits, accomplishing things that most people do not. He is said to have always been very hands-on in his business dealings and is extremely altruistic, overcoming obstacles with ease while inspiriting others to do the same.

He married former model Ivana Zelnickova in 1977, with whom he had three children: Donald Jr, Ivanka, and Eric. Living a very high-profile life, Trump constantly garnered interest from press and tabloids, after which the couple divorced in 1992 and he married actress Marla Maples. Marla gave birth to daughter Tiffany Trump in 1993 and later, Donald Trump married his current wife, model and former First Lady Melania Knauss, to whom their son Barron was born in 2006.

Trump often mused at running for president when speaking in interviews, and eventually announced his candidacy in the 2016 U.S. presidential election.

Although at first glance he was an obvious outsider and underdog, his candid personality gained him millions of supporters. Americans were not used to hearing direct communication of his ideas and emotions in the political arena using social media tools such as Twitter.

Trump applied his skills as a tough businessman, real estate developer, bestselling author and popular television personality and parlayed them into the political arena.

He ran against former Secretary of State and former First Lady Hillary Clinton in 2016, which featured debates unlike anything the electorate had seen before. Like him or not, Trump projected a presence and an uncanny way about him that drew attention on the presidential debate stage.

Although Trump received no endorsements from major newspapers—long regarded as essential to election victory, his confidence, humor and toughness pulled him through, and he won the majority of the Electoral College, making his win one of the biggest political upsets in modern American history.

JOHN FITZGERALD KENNEDY JR.

John Fitzgerald Kennedy Jr., born November 25, 1960 was the handsome and charismatic son of iconic President John F. Kennedy and his elegant wife, America's First Lady Jacqueline Kennedy. He lived in the White House during the first three years of his life along with older sister Caroline until his father was ruthlessly assassinated in 1963. America still vividly remembers John as a young boy faithfully and chillingly saluting his slain father's casket.

JFK Jr. grew up in the public spotlight. People were fascinated with him. Paparazzi trailed his every move but he handled the paparazzi and press with grace, charm and patience. He had a dazzling smile and oozed charisma. He could even turn it on or off at will when he did or didn't want to be noticed.

He was handsome, humble, witty and possessed great character and virtues. He was a clever man who became a lawyer, a journalist and publisher of his own magazine he called George. He had even worked as a New York assistant district attorney for nearly four years.

He vowed to find out who murdered his father even if he had to take the whole government apart. There are even rumors that this clever man had the chutzpah to fake his own death, had a family with Carolyn out of the spotlight and has been doing what he had vowed to do.

America always had a warm spot for the Kennedy dynasty and John was undisputedly known as the prince of Camelot. He was even picked by People magazine in 1988 as the Sexiest Man Alive.

John met his stylish and charismatic future wife Carolyn Bessette in 1994 when she was a publicist for Calvin Klein. He soon married her at a secret ceremony in 1996 but their young lives as well as Carolyn's sister, Lauren, were cut short when they died in that fateful plane crash off Martha's Vineyard in 1999. John was so loved by America that he had even been declared the front runner for the New York Senate seat before his untimely death.

SCOTT HARRISON

You may be wondering if the only way your charisma can shine is to have an incredible talent, a great bit of luck, or, in the case of Malala, a great bit of adversity to fall on you. Do you need any of these to find the charisma factor in yourself and to be able to use it for the good of others and humankind? Well, it's very simply not the case. Giants walk among us every day, brushing by us in the street, and we may not even realize what lies just under their veneers.

Take a case in point with Scott Harrison, who is by some standards a rather ordinary fellow who grew up in the suburban world of New Jersey. He found and used his incredible charisma factor to make remarkable changes in this world.

Born September 7, 1975, Harrison later worked as a New York City nightclub and party promoter throwing lavish events for the likes of Elle magazine, major fashion houses, VH1, MTV, and Bacardi. He made tons of cool party friends but felt his life was vapid—he even described himself as "the worst person I knew." Quitting his job, he volunteered as a photojournalist on the Mercy Ships taking trips to Liberia in Africa to provide free health care to those that needed it most. What he saw there was to change his destiny and direction forever, and fortunately also to change the destiny for literally millions of others.

Scott noticed that a deplorable lack of fresh water was the root cause of most disease in Liberia. He knew he had to use what he had to try to set it right. He brought back pictures of people that he had taken during his two years on the ships to all of those old night-clubbing friends of his in New York and staged some big, charity-style events like he used to in his life before the Mercy Ship. What came out of these events is today one of the leading organizations providing water in the continent.

Scott has truly found his calling. When he speaks in front of an audience about his charity and his mission, one sees his charisma and passion leaping out of his pores. Why?

Because he loves what he does from his core. His charisma, charity work, and desire to make things better for others have become one with his existence. So, next time you tell yourself "I can't really make a mark, because I'm not a celebrity" or "I haven't had anything extraordinary happen to me," think again. A humble kid from New Jersey did it, and changed millions of lives for the better.

Using your personal charisma factor for the good of others and the betterment of the world pays you back ten times over. You will watch others become drawn to your charismatic self as you grow by leaps you never thought imaginable.

CHARLIE CHAPLIN

Also known as "the Little Tramp", Charlie Chaplin has given immense happiness and amusement to audiences throughout the world. He had such a charisma factor that his comedy films remain immortal many years after his death.

The comedy legend was born Charles Spencer Chaplin in London. A gem of the silent film era, he had the power to make people understand what he wanted to convey through his body language and simple clothing. His whole body acted, not just his face and hands, and he made people laugh endlessly. He created legendary characters that few other comedians have surpassed. Apart from being a comic actor and live stage comedian, he was a film director and, at times, also filled the role of composer.

The secret of Chaplin's charisma was not in his acting and comic skills; it was rather in his ability to transform inner silence and sadness into laughter and amusement. It really requires charisma to hide pain, and it requires strength to convert dark and dense pain into something beautiful and positive. That's what Chaplin did, and that's the reason the whole world remembers him, continues to learn things from his personality, and tries to adopt the principle of converting pain into something better and beautiful. I personally adore his work.

If you can illuminate your inner charisma factor and look at the brighter side of life, you can certainly fight troubles and negativity. You might not be famous like Chaplin or any other Hollywood star, but you would be happy in your own world and have the strength to maintain your happiness. All it takes is a combination of effort, honesty, energy, and dedication to discover the charisma within you. Even those who are born with it in abundance must do a lot to protect it, maintain it, and keep it shining.

ANDY WARHOL

Art has its own charisma, which is why many artists are charismatic. They have something different in them that just isn't commonly found. It can stem from their specialty within art or their sense of creativity, power of imagination, or confidence in creating something new. Born Andrew Warhola in Pittsburgh, Pennsylvania, in 1928, Warhol's art even has its own museum in his native city. He is still one of the most esteemed names in art, thirty-four years after his death in 1987.

Warhol's charisma factor rested in the versatility of the artwork he offered to the world. He was a multitasker and came up with many ideas at the same time. Above all, he had the strength to execute them and bring them to the world in material form. He was not only famous for his general art but also for pioneering the concept of computer-based art. His compositions in hand drawing, painting, printmaking, photography, silk-screening, sculpture, film, and music reflect the essence of the magnetism he held within himself. He was known as one of the finest and most polished artists, holding the charm to change the world effectively.

Andy Warhol upgraded the existing levels of art in all those different forms. His is a leading name in the Pop Art movement, and anyone who visits the museum that bears his name will find exclusive artistic creations reflecting his essence and excellence. Warhol held the charisma factor of his artistic sense and new ideas from his imagination. At the same time, he was strong enough to pursue his ideas and keep them alive even after his own life ended.

Since I have studied numerous charismatic personalities, including Warhol, I strongly believe that the charisma factor within you is not only a thing of charm and brilliance but also a responsibility. Being fully engaged in performing your duties and chasing your goals passionately keeps the charisma factor alive in you.

MICHAEL JACKSON

As the distressing news of the death of an American pop sensation began to circulate on June 25, 2009, the whole world turned melancholy. Yahoo, AOL, Google, and other search engines crashed as millions of Internet users hit the search button to find out whether it was true. Fans who were praying this was some kind of prank were disappointed when television news channels as well as major Internet news sites confirmed that Michael Jackson was no more.

The moonwalker, charismatic singer, and enthusiastic composer who was born in 1958 was laid to rest in Los Angeles, but he still shines like a star in the hearts of millions of his fans. Throughout his successful career as a pop star, he appeared in this world like live magic, entering straight into the hearts of people and making a special place for himself. Like other celebrities, he went through traumatizing times amid allegations of sexual abuse and other controversies. But that didn't hamper his star power, his onstage image, or the special power within him, which remained untouched. Apart from his talent, his dedication, and his supreme sense for pop music, he had the charisma factor, which remains alive in the hearts of many.

Despite his artificially carved face, Jackson had an attractive personality and a wide appeal. Fans loved his appearance, including his feminine moves, and would do anything to listen to his songs. As an example, the posthumously released film, *This Is It,* was nominated for and won several awards.

Jackson had the charisma factor as an artist; his belief in his art was his strength, and he was known as the King of Pop. His songs and live stage performances made people move and groove. He was the ideal for many people—they approved of his never-ending energy and power to perform with passion. Jackson lived his passion from the core, something he taught the world through his music. Those who had questions in their minds about what made him so unique could only be answered with the word charisma.

Learn to develop your own unique sense of style and hone your talents. Michael Jackson knew he was a talented composer, singer, and dancer, and he dedicated much of his time to becoming the best performer he could possibly be. Hard work and true talent can set you apart from the rest of the crowd.

NELSON MANDELA

Known throughout South Africa by his very respected clan name of Madiba, Nelson Mandela, former president of South Africa

(1994 to 1999), was the first democratically elected president of the country. Trained as a lawyer, in his early days he was an activist with the African National Congress and founded the Umkhonto we Sizwe, which was an armed wing of the party. He was an advocate for peaceful change and dedicated his life to a fight against apartheid in his country. He detested racialism, because he regarded it as a barbaric thing, whether it came from a black man or a white man.

The man who lived twenty-seven years of his life in prison has been rightly called the Tata, which in Xhosa, his native language, means "father."

He strove for justice and truth at all levels throughout his life. His book, Long Walk to Freedom, was more than a thousand pages filled with this passion and drive. When his son died of AIDS, Mandela used the opportunity to speak out about the AIDS problem rather than follow the government line, which at that time did not even acknowledge the fact that AIDS existed.

This man's charisma was derived from his rich life experiences, from his birth on July 18, 1918, to his recent death in December 2013. That is correct: he had a life of ninety-five years, with little time wasted, which is why his presence was still felt in world politics up to and beyond his death. His spirit will live forever, and South Africa will always be grateful to him. He gave it an identity as well as freedom. That freedom had a cost: violence came when his peaceful effort produced no results. It certainly took its toll in the form of lives lost and years of Mandela's own liberty taken. His stoicism and dedication to his principles meant he was willing to give up twenty-seven long years of his life to win the emancipation of his people.

His compassion and generosity are two of the primary factors that made him so charismatic. He realized early in life that thoughts of violence would only add to the prevailing hatred in the whole of Africa. To him, the only way to win back the freedom his country lacked was to embrace love and forgiveness.

One thing Mandela learned in prison, which became the motivating factor of his life, was to discard hatred and distress for the good of all. Kindness and care are the most significant elements that can unite people. This association helps everyone to work toward the common goal of achieving freedom. In fact, this is what he taught the entire world as soon as he was released from prison. This is what his life's ideology depended on and what made him a true father who thinks of everyone and was willing to help all without a second thought. This was his underlying meaning when he said, "I dream of an Africa which is in peace with itself."

Nelson Mandela was an extraordinary example of the seamless blending of charisma and strong, noble personal ideals. He won the adoration of his people, and there were few global leaders that were not present among the throngs of adoring South Africans as he was laid to rest.

MAHATMA GANDHI

Nelson Mandela and Martin Luther King, Jr. were both inspired by the same person: Mohandas Karamchand Gandhi, the man who taught India to fight with grace and nonviolence. This epitome of charisma was born in 1869 and was assassinated in 1948. This is what he had to say against violence of any kind, which he would not tolerate: "An eye for an eye will only make the whole world blind." Not only did he assist India to unify but also led a march against the British salt taxes. His civil disobedience, marches, and, finally, the Quit India movement, paved the way for Indian independence. Yes, there were a lot of factors and people who contributed in small and big ways to win this freedom, but Mahatma Gandhi played a central role.

His ability to connect to the masses instantly and at their level was the most remarkable element of his charismatic personality. It is true that no one else in the history of Indian politics has ever been able to command the multitudes as he could. He had always been a person of great repute; even the British couldn't help but give in to his demands, as they were so polite in nature. Nonviolence was the path he chose for expressing his difference of opinion. He taught the Indian people to have faith in themselves and follow a path of honesty. Integrity and determination were two of the most important elements he found were required to achieve anything great. There is no need to explain that this worked in favor of India and its people.

Not just anyone comes to be considered the father of a nation. Gandhi proved himself the only person who could guide India in a positive way. He combined traditional sentiments with modern values to shape a new country. He was never a show-off and always kept wealth at bay because he found truth to be the most powerful aspect of life. The best part about his charisma is that he never imposed himself; instead, he observed and learned different things from different scenarios. His varied experiences strengthened his values.

His charismatic personality could enchant the masses much like a hypnotic charm that helped people to unite and listen to him. The spirit of his ideology still lingers in the world, which makes him eternal. In the words of Albert Einstein,

"Generations to come will scarce believe that such a one as this ever in flesh and blood walked upon this earth".

Ahimsa is the practice of nonviolence toward all living beings. Gandhi stood for it; I practice it as well, as I have all my life. The more you practice it, the more compassionate you will become and the more you will develop empathy for others and can relate to them better.

The individuals just discussed are among the most charismatic people in history, fully emblematic of what it means to live a life expressive of charisma's power. Now, consider your own path. Which of their traits would you most like to learn to emulate? Which of their passions echo your own? How can you turn inspiration into action, and motivation into results?

Chapter 6

Can You Create Charisma?

We all want to be liked and loved, but what gets others to like and love us? Do you have something special in you that people recognize and really appreciate? Do you feel eyes following you as you move through life, not staring but offering you glances of appreciation?

"Charisma to me is when someone attracts people because of their personality and warmth and they light up the room. You either have it or you don't," says Housewives of New York City star Ramona Singer.

Charisma is a way of seeing and perceiving things, a sort of magnetism that inspires adoration and confidence—like charm, luck, reputation, and influence, which all may draw attention to us. The effort you put into being likable matters a lot. A little inner voice may say, "But I don't have that type of personality" or "I am what I am; how can I change myself?" It's true that you are what you are, but the question is, are you the best you can be?

Developing your charisma factor isn't about changing yourself; it's about developing yourself with a strong belief: "Yes, I can, and yes, I will." It's about imagining, practicing, and moving toward your new charismatic self. Often people are amazed to find that they can change what they think they can't. Why do you think you can't create charisma in yourself? Are those who hold magnificent charms of positivity also human beings like you? Yes! They're very much like you, but what makes them stand out is the eternal faith they possess for whatever they have in their personality. They consider it a gift from the supreme power, nurture it with their acts of positivity, and retain it with full determination.

The discovery of your charisma begins with believing in yourself and inner motivation, which is already resting deep within you. All you require is to clear any psychological and physical barriers that keep you from believing in yourself. This will bring you out of your comfort zone. You must overcome all the negative beliefs, apprehensions, fears, and doubts. Discard any negativity that may have been breeding in you for a long time. This will mean beginning a lifelong process of contemplation that requires your complete dedication and honesty. And finally, after discovering the precious and priceless gift of the charisma factor, it becomes your prime responsibility to protect and maintain it. Rome was not built in a day. You also can't create or discover the spark in you in a day.

The urge to discover your charisma is strongest when you observe charismatic people around you and you see them spreading their magic, when their irresistible charm speaks louder than their words. When their magnetism attracts everyone around them. The magnetism of someone's charismatic presence around you makes you yearn to be like that person, and you are mesmerized by the thought of the level of prosperity he or she enjoys by being charismatic. The desire to catch the power of this charisma is too fascinating to be escaped.

The beautiful and vibrant shine of charisma rests in every individual soul; the only need is to wake it up and make it bloom so that the whole world can see your arresting inner beauty, which is charisma itself. Being human, you need to realize the power you have of creating charisma in yourself. The mistake that most people make is to try to find the source and cause of charisma in the outer world, however, it lies within. The common person has to realize that charisma is not anyone's special privilege; even they can achieve virtually anything they want or desire. Becoming charismatic is not only an arbitrary gift of God. If you want to be charismatic, you can be, you just need to realize your inner urge and inner spark, which can flourish—and with flying colors once it does.

Charisma can be thought of as one's inner resting beauty, but one has to understand how to nurture it. There are several techniques for discovering the hidden charm in every individual. Once you focus on the methods, reaching the zenith of charm and spark becomes possible, but it's not easy. You need to fully dedicate and devote yourself to the purpose of finding the brighter and better side of you. All you need to do is to learn and perceive how to maximize the value of your assets and to deploy them so that you not only attract people but also keep them hooked.

The techniques for boosting your charisma factor can give you the power to do all tasks efficiently and effectively. They can be the key to success and growth in everything, whether in the personal or social realms. We all are unique, infinitely creative human beings. Each of us has something unique and special to offer that no one else can. We just have to identify and develop our unique characteristics. They can work as a magnetic force for you, grabbing the attention of people around you. Charisma is not only learned, but is an acquired capability that is later refined with experience and allows the persona to flourish.

Does charisma come automatically, or does it develop when we identify that we need it? Does it have anything to do with our upbringing? Is it built in and only in need of polishing our inner strength? Well, there is only one answer to all these questions: every one of us is born with uniqueness and a special quality called charisma. We need only to identify it and nurture it so that we can display it to the masses.

Some think people are born with it, and some think they must develop it. Those who realize they are born with charisma can influence from the very beginning. As time passes, it develops further, which results in a charismatic personality. Those who only later identify a need to develop charisma become introspective and find their hidden beauty. This becomes their charisma and all the charm and spark associated with it.

When we encounter charismatic personalities, we recognize our need for charisma.

Upbringing has some impact on charisma, but it largely depends on how someone perceives it later. Charisma is inborn. It is always there somewhere, at the bottom of every personality. Once people identify it, the gains associated with it follow.

Charisma is not something that only well-known personalities own. We can all think of countless famous personalities who do not have charisma (or do not reflect their charismatic sides).

There are several techniques for developing incredible charisma that are extremely powerful. They require one to be at the pinnacle of physical and emotional fitness, as the intensity needed for developing this skill is higher than that needed for anything else. Once this state is established, positive energy will be created. Ultimately, this aura can make you more charismatic for an entire day or even for several days. But you should practice regularly to achieve the best result of these techniques: an ultimately charismatic personality, the personality you find to have a strange attractiveness, the personality that has all the power to influence and persuade others, the personality that leads others naturally in thought, action, and perception. See the workbook.

Every person has potential charisma hidden in him or her. It may be dormant, but it can become active the moment it is discovered. Some do not even know that it exists in them until they face situations that make them realize it does. Many, in fact, think too much about what they should have done but were not able to. However, many people live according to how they think they should, although life should not be lived on assumptions. The lives of these people flow with their thoughts, experiences, and learning. They try to display their best selves to everyone, but instead of focusing on who you think you should be, you should focus on who you are. We sometimes disconnect from who we actually are when we meet a charismatic personality because we are so influenced by their charm.

What can we project as our best asset? How can we best fulfill our potential? What is our true power? What is our core potential? How can we improve? We try very hard to be alike and to imitate others, but this just distracts us from the bottom line: charisma radiates from you when you have the strength and courage to be yourself. Charisma reflects when you believe in your own potential and expand it to its best. Interestingly, we admire those who have the courage to be themselves, those who make us believe and follow them.

People appreciate the charismatic because they appreciate themselves. Charismatic people have the courage to be who they really are. They project the best parts of themselves. They are very much familiar not only with their strengths and weaknesses, but also with their own uniqueness and their own spark. This is the foundation on which their personality has been built.

When we love and accept our inner selves, we begin with the process of self-realization—then charisma will follow naturally. Our self-esteem is the power that builds our personalities, defines who we really are, and provides an ideal inner aura for developing the qualities of charisma. We just need to identify this self-esteem; ultimately, it is about finding yourself. Override your negative thoughts with positive ones.

Many people spend their entire lives dreaming about being someone else instead of realizing their real selves are within them. Once you identify yours, no one can attack you. This will leave you with extraordinary power—of being yourself, of being charismatic. You just need to identify your power. Ask yourself right now why you need someone or something to trigger bringing the best out of yourself. Look at your workplace, for example. Why do some people not perform at their best until and unless they are under extreme pressure to do it? Why do many people who are good at many things—and know they are—need someone to notice it? Everyone wants his or her work to be noticed, but why expect your inner beauty to be noticed by someone else?

The answers to these questions rests in you. Come up with the new you and expose and surprise the world by exposing the best of yourself to the whole world. Why not let everybody recognize and appreciate you? This is only possible if you explore yourself better first. When someone is close to you, like your parents, siblings, or spouse, you can expect them to identify the spark in you, but when you wait for them to notice it before you groom it, it is a waste of your time and life. You need to think differently, don't think thoughts that make you suffer or put substances into your body, which aren't easily processed.

Charisma is a strange feeling of confidence. That makes you feel alive. It is a pleasing communication with the world. Charisma brings along with it several perks and benefits that, when people observe them, they have an urge to achieve as well. When we observe charismatic people and see how people are affected by their presence and the degree of attention and love they receive, we crave charisma too.

Take President Donald Trump, for example. When we observe the degree of joy that he experiences in being charismatic from huge crowds who listen to him, we imagine ourselves in his place.

Charismatic people have the extraordinary ability to attract people. Their body language speaks louder than words. Their confidence is reflected in each step they take. They deal well with adverse people and situations. We can even learn charismatic behavior from autobiographies and life histories of many charismatic characters. Apart from the famous personalities, though, we can learn charismatic behavior from anyone whom we observe and feel positive and magnetic vibes from.

Charismatic people exude a degree of magic that has an extraordinary power to change any situation to their favor with their powers. They know how to convert the opposing tide toward them. They know how to make the best out of any situation. They know how to deal with opposition and criticism. Their lives seem to be full of wonderful opportunities and possibilities. It is something that each of us has a right to have and to feel. Why waste our best opportunity? Live life fully. Give a return gift to the Almighty by living every moment to the fullest extent. Praise yourself for getting it and living it. Your charisma will emerge as a beautiful ray of sunlight that is full of hope and expectation for what life has to offer. Very soon, people will gather around you and will look to you to find out what makes you so charismatic and so successful!

Chapter 7

What Are the Qualities of Charismatic People?

Charisma is the culmination of many qualities. As we've learned, charisma is the positive energy inside you that you need to channel in the right ways. This positive energy could be your passion, your dedication, or it could even be your wish to learn things. All these are positives of a character that may help form a charismatic personality if properly developed.

EXPERTS OF THE GAME

According to Max Weber, the renowned anthropologist and sociologist, charisma is "a certain quality" in the personality that is achieved "by virtue", virtue that sets you apart from others. A charismatic person exhibits some extraordinary qualities that makes him or her the equivalent of someone with "exceptional powers or qualities", Weber further elucidates. So, this, again, implies that charisma should be used positively to produce the desired effect.

A BEHAVIORAL STUDY

You may have heard about charisma the way a neuro-linguistic programming (NLP) study describes it. Let's look at behavioral patterns of charismatic personalities. (Though, naturally, people react differently to situations.) NLP is a system of alternative therapy that aids in self-awareness and examines and analyzes how some people can outperform others at the same task. Those who excel are sometimes recognized as charismatic.

THE COMPARISON

Charismatic personalities differ from one another. This shouldn't surprise you, because a charismatic personality is also a human being, and no two people are completely alike. For example, if we compare Dr. Martin Luther King, Jr. with Muhammad Ali, two of the most charismatic personalities of their times and beyond, we clearly see huge differences between them. One is a boxer and the other was a Noble Peace Prize recipient. They couldn't possibly be the same. They had different body languages, and Dr. King was an accomplished orator, while Ali was soft-spoken outside the ring.

Margaret Thatcher, known as the Iron Lady, used eye contact with her oratorical skills as a weapon to assert herself and prove a point. If you look at the way President Trump addresses the public, even today, he uses smiles as his weapons as well as timely pauses. Prince William and Duchess Kate are charismatic personalities whose charismas are balanced, and they use them to influence people in the best possible ways.

Charisma varies from person to person. Charisma can be

thought of as the art of impressing people, and dedicating oneself to the service of the community can enhance it. That means one needs to express the desire to serve a larger group by paying attention to them above one's own interests. This aspiration inevitably releases a positive energy, which will influence people all the more.

THE RELATIVITY OF CHARISMA

Charisma is contextual. That is to say, charismatic people can spin it around themselves whenever they want and let it go when it's not required. Many examples establish this point. During a shopping spree Marilyn Monroe went with one of her close friends, no one noticed that the star who could set the screen on fire was in their midst. However, when she shed her cloak of concealment, she was immediately mobbed.

THE IMPORTANCE OF CHARM

Charisma has to come from within. One can't be charismatic until one actually feels it. People have to blend the goodness of charisma and positive thinking into their characters consciously. Charismatic people don't use only external tools like body language and sweet talk. These are people who stand out and can influence our thoughts. They have some sort of brilliance about them. Again, charisma can't be faked. It might be possible to fool one, two, three, or ten people, but no more than that. Fake charisma can't bring the multitudes together to carry out a task. For that, one has to be really charming and possess true charisma.

Charisma should be used in a reassuring way that gives people hope. This reassurance, in turn, will make people believe in you. The hope will support your cause, as people know you aren't deviating from the path of honesty. Again, people only put their trust in you if they know you have faith in yourself. This is a harmonious chain reaction that flows smoothly from one thought to another. Although thoughts are anchored in the mind, they flow freely in both directions—to and from you. Only then will your public speaking have the desired impact on others, and people will be enticed to follow you. You'll find that your communications are effective, and all your hard work pays off.

THE ART OF CHARISMA

Before we continue, we need to discuss a few additional things that make up charisma. Again, we aren't talking about looking good—there are plenty of charismatic people who aren't handsome or beautiful. It's not about wearing particular clothes or an expensive perfume, what parties you go to or how much money you have. It's purely your personality and the inner beauty of your soul that are reflected in your charisma. When you're in touch with the beauty that rests deep within you, you will be vested with all the power you need to remain true to yourself.

Let's take a look at the elements that constitute the complete package of charisma.

Self-confidence. Are you really happy with yourself? If the answer is yes, then you surely don't need to put up a false front and pretend you're someone else. Knowing you're self-sufficient and able to solve all the mysteries of your life makes all the difference in the world. In fact, you can boost the confidence of and offer encouragement to others.

The gaze. Maintaining eye contact is one of the most important things for a charismatic personality to do. It's rightly said that your eyes are the mirrors to your inner self, and you can be sure that if you look people in the eye, they'll know exactly what you mean. It's as if your soul is trying to connect with theirs, and that's how your charm casts a spell on them.

It should be soft and not prolonged. This gaze will make them comfortable and will lead to people wanting to strike up a conversation with you.

This moment. When you talk with people, be present in the moment, making them feel there's no one else in the room other than the two of you. This indicates that you're paying attention to what someone is saying. This is the moment when you can sweep people off their feet with your charisma the way President Clinton does. Of course, you would feel the same way if people listened with their utmost attention to what you were saying.

Successful listening. It's rightly said that it is very hard to find listeners in this world. So, if you are present in the moment and listening to others, you have an audience. When people are done talking, they want to listen to you. A good listener always wins the case, so if you want to be a public figure, you know that you have to listen. Only then can you truly understand others' problems. You can then try to find solutions, even if it takes time to think of them.

Effective communication. You want your audiences to be spellbound. Show enthusiasm. Make your speeches interesting. And don't ignore the need to be interesting while talking to people one on one. That's a challenge, and you'll need to put in a lot of practice time on it. Add humor to your words, and always focus on the positive. Never speak ill of others in public or talk about what you don't like or other negative things. Your aura of positivity will make you different from the rest. Most of us complain quite a bit.

All these practices will definitely help you make your presence felt in a room full of people. It happens slowly but steadily and will change you forever. Don't rush into things or create a fake charismatic personality to try to get it to happen right away. You'll be caught red-handed if you just put on an act, leading to possible public humiliation. That's something we won't discuss here. Let's continue to focus on the positive. (See the workbook for more practical tools to develop these skills).

Chapter 8

Charisma in Business

To be the charismatic leader that everyone looks to for guidance and direction in any work setting, you need to realize that charisma is an art just like dancing, singing, or painting. That means you need to learn it first and then hone it to perfection. You need to work diligently to develop it and then make it gel with your personality.

Charisma can also be described as your behavior toward others. It has to be adjusted according to the people with whom you are communicating. Charisma is like a jargon that others can understand. Speaking in the appropriate way will help you in your career as well as in your personal growth.

There is a specific protocol for developing charisma in any situation at work or in your social life that will pay off in spades:

- **Body language.** Always stand straight, without slouching. Don't cross your legs or arms while seated, and look people in the eye while speaking. Show your confidence.

- **Smile.** As already mentioned, a warm smile will make others feel comfortable in your presence.
- **Look like a leader.** Speak with every person on your team, and make him or her want to work harder by boosting his or her enthusiasm. Your grooming and outward appearance must also be appropriate to the message you want to convey.

Take, for example, at First Lady Melania Trump. Every one of her outfits is carefully selected to respect and be appropriate to each event she attends. While charisma is not a beauty contest, to underestimate the power of your outward appearance only sells short what you want to deliver. If you're with a large group, speak clearly and sensibly about topics everyone can relate to. Add humor to instill a sense of camaraderie in your audience and win them over to your message.

PERSONAL DEVELOPMENT AND THE WORKPLACE

A charming and engaging personality will help you in all aspects of your life, not the least of which is to make a real impression in the boardroom and work setting. Work is not just about the skills and knowledge you bring to the table. It is also about constantly engaging with others to successfully sell your ideas. If you bring a charming personality to work, you will achieve things that others cannot.

Your personality is formed from your value system. It's a reflection of the background from which you came and the conditions in which you grew up. Then, development also forms a part of your personality as you continue to learn. Education and enlightenment have always been considered great ways to develop your personality.

You can find many self-help books on personality development. You can read case studies and integrate their suggestions into your own life. You can find personality tests on the Internet or read books to learn more about your personality type. However, always maintain your own personal value system. There is no point in making yourself into something that you do not genuinely feel from the gut. Everyone easily spots a false personality, a fake.

Then, of course, you can continue to refine your personality to make it a better fit for the work setting and even the social circles you expect to join.

If your personality is already well evolved, your personal charisma factor will only enhance it, helping you in your personal and business lives.

INSPIRING AND LEADING WITH WORDS

Words of encouragement can help you inspire other colleagues and staff. In social situations, they always help you make friends.

Here are some points to remember:

- Choose your words carefully to convey respect for others.
- Learn the skill of negotiation through words. Sometimes it is what you don't say that may win the battle.
- Influence people by truly listening. Then respond with caring and empathetic words.
- Encourage those who are younger than you, or those that look up to you in a work setting, to respect you

by truly helping them with words of encouragement and wisdom.

WORKING TOWARD INDIVIDUAL AND PROFESSIONAL GROWTH

Self-awareness. To grow, you need to have self-awareness. Be conscious about your choices and reactions. You need to have a clear understanding of your behavior and thought processes. Focus on details of your behavior and personality.

Relationships. Maintaining good personal and professional relationships is important. Handle all your relationships delicately and honestly. There is a saying in business: "never burn your bridges". You never know who might be helpful to you in achieving your career goals and dreams.

Proficiencies. When we talk about business skills, we think only of how they apply to business—strategy building, networking, innovative thinking, team handling, supervising, creating new products, making sales, and getting the pitch right. All this competence can be useful in your personal life as well. Make maximum use of your resources.

Practice. The saying "Practice makes perfect" is true. In today's highly competitive world, it's the only way to remain a front-runner. Honing and developing your delivery skills are crucial to your career and you need to keep at them. In the present age of global businesses, employers look for abilities that may not be easy to include on your résumé. Let them shine in interviews—or you risk not getting that new job you know you are perfect for. For example, acquiring new clients is a key to successful business in any area.

Hone your skills and be able to demonstrate them. Show employers that you can:

- Gain clients' confidence by meeting their demands
- Analyze requirements
- Be a good listener and ask questions that lead to better understanding
- Be flexible and change according to the demands of any situation
- Provide quality, steady work

If you think you're too busy to do all this, you need to rethink and work on that attitude. Developing a charismatic business personality is often as crucial to your success as the skills you bring to the table.

"When Leesa asked me for my thoughts on the topic of charisma, I immediately visualized the "who" in charismatic," quips reality television personality Lisa Gastineau.

"Who is this person that exudes charisma? My gut reaction is a person who brings positivity and light to their surroundings," she continues. "When you speak of charisma, it varies in opinion, similar to beauty. Everyone has a different ideal of what is beautiful in their eyes. The un- quenchable "it" factor. For me, I've concluded that these 4 Cs hold the magic of charisma, in no particular order: charm, confidence, captivation and composure.

"The perfect combination of confidence mixed with a strong dose of humbleness. Not arrogant, egotistical or frazzled. Charm and confidence flow easily from the charismatic individual, since it comes from merit, not ego. There is a confident way they are able to address a group, yet have you feel they are talking directly to you and your soul.

"In reality, charisma is a gift—but it's one which can be attained by all. I personally feel that when I need to address a group—whether it's giving a motivational speech or selling my jewelry on Home Shopping TV—the longer I pause and plan, the better it prepares me to be my best.

"My armor, as I like to call it," Lisa confides. "From the clothes and jewelry I wear, down to the critical information I need to know to create my confidence. It takes planning to accomplish, but it's what gives me the ability to project positive feelings."

Charismatic people have a way to communicate that creates a form of unity. They make people want to believe what they say, without question.

"When I create jewelry for my Lisa Gastineau collection, I always keep in mind that certain gemstones have properties—believed for centuries to have the ability to make you tap into your inner strength, beauty and confidence," Lisa adds with enthusiasm.

"You can bet that I am always wearing them, as are many of my clients who trust me to help them find their perfect pieces. For example, aquamarine is the stone I wear when I need to communicate.

In charisma, there is no room for self-doubt. When you believe in yourself, it shows—in a positive, charismatic way."

Now that you know so much about charismatic personality, work toward yours by going after better opportunities. You can earn a fortune with the right mix of characteristics. Have you ever wondered why you got passed up for a promotion? Failed to get a job that you believed you were perfect for?

Pitched a project, only to have the prospect decide to go with another firm? There are often many causes of such events, but if you look carefully and honestly, you may find that a truly charismatic individual took the prize that you wanted. A charismatic person flourishes more than the others around him or her.

CHARISMATIC LEADERS

Many people want to lead, but they fail because they don't have the right skills or haven't yet developed their strengths. Charisma is all about doing things right, and you need to have the aptitude for leadership to succeed. Focus on your strong points and cultivate them. Here are a few pointers that can help you to become a good charismatic leader over time:

- Keep long-term goals in mind. A leader remains focused on the big picture
- Be realistic and able to troubleshoot all kinds of problems
- Be confident enough to take risks when required
- Take a strong stand when necessary
- Communicate effectively
- Understand people and work with them in harmony
- Lead from the front
- Be visionary
- Inspire and motivate others
- Show confidence and boost others' morale
- Be energetic. Your enthusiasm will inspire others

- Be a subject matter expert with the ability to think outside the box.

All these qualities can make charismatic leaders. They are captivating people who are referred to as doers and achievers. They inspire others to follow them and are always in great demand.

Chapter 9

Charisma and Performance

I want to share with you a bit about how the charisma factor is important in my line of work. Perhaps my thoughts can shed some light, no matter your chosen field or path. I doubt that I would have been chosen for any of the roles I've played if I hadn't emphasized developing the presence I hold within. I am a vulnerable and highly sensitive person. I think you have to be in this business.

There are innumerable talented actors out there, but few have that extra-special something. People who don't want to explore their charisma can certainly sit in the audience and applaud for the ones who want to know about it.

Charisma is a magical power that makes an audience hold its breath as it watches a performer. The audience, mesmerized by the performer's charms, can't look away. Every performer wants to achieve finesse and wants spectators to react this way. It gives them aesthetic satisfaction and allows them even more roles to choose from as the demand for their skills increases.

To make a performance memorable for the audience, a

performer needs to practice his or her art regularly, in the same way practicing charisma is necessary. Performers need to be charismatic if they really want to make themselves appealing to spectators. No one likes to buy tickets for a boring show. What do you, as an audience member, hope to achieve by attending a movie in a theater? The answer is obvious: you want to be entertained. But if the movie doesn't have a good cast or an interesting story line, you won't bother to see it.

A movie featuring Mel Gibson, Kate Winslet, Robin Williams, Cameron Diaz or Dustin Hoffman might titillate your desire sufficiently, perhaps based entirely on the draw of those names alone. And why do these actors interest you? A common response is that they exude charisma, which gets us, the viewers, to stay in our seats. We're captivated every time they appear on-screen with their magnetism and talent—that very magical something that draws us to watch them.

The connection between the performers and audience puts us in a trance-like state that steals us away from reality as we relate to the fictional characters. This relationship amuses us and makes us feel good

THE TRUTH ABOUT CHARISMATIC PERFORMERS

A charismatic entertainer has a lot of responsibilities to pay attention to. Charismatic people know this fact very well, because they have already connected to their inner selves. They enjoy challenging themselves and going the extra mile, which indicates that they're free to experiment with their talent, learning new things, changing the way they look, and setting trends. Trendsetting is an area where charismatic personalities never fall short. Think of Taylor Swift, Kanye West, or Michael Jackson.

This sets them apart from the rest of the world, as they are ready for all sorts of challenges. They have to overcome fear of all kinds to do what they do. Fear limits us and sets boundaries, but charismatic people know how to transcend them. They realize that the bottom line is the need to cultivate their charisma, and they are smart enough to know that no matter how demanding that may be, that to not embrace it and to utilize it to the best of their abilities will only sell their skills and their careers short. To quote Swami Vivekananda, "Be not afraid of anything. You will do marvelous work. It is fear that is the great cause of misery in the world. It is fear that is the greatest of all superstitions. It is fear that is the cause of all our woes, and it is fearlessness that brings heaven even in a moment. Therefore, 'arise, awake and stop not until the goal is reached.'"

Charismatic entertainers generally act in a controlled manner and maintain decency in public. They may feel compelled to do so because they're constantly on the radar. They need to keep a grip on themselves that others don't. Remember, many of these charismatic personalities are role models for society. They have to be sensible, at least while under public scrutiny. For well-known stars, any move they make without keeping their behavior in check has the potential to spell disaster. Even highly charismatic people can have bad days.

Another fact about charisma is that it isn't necessarily related to intelligence. This may be an astonishing revelation. Clearly, intelligence isn't the only characteristic that arouses the masses. That's why we're so disappointed when our favorite celebrities do something foolish. It may be reassuring to know that you don't have to be a genius to succeed, but you still need some common sense or intelligence.

Honing your charisma can cover up the fact that you don't have a law degree from Harvard. Often, people say that all you need to do is focus on one or two top qualities or top skills and play them up for all they are worth. They become your ace cards. You don't have to have an entire deck, just play your ace cards along with your well-honed charisma, and you will likely find success.

You probably differ from your loved ones over who is the best in any field. The fact is that charismatic personalities are all different. While you may try to identify each person's charisma, even personalities from the same trade have different charismatic appeal. We've already discussed how the charisma factor differs from person to person.

Just like a performer's, your skills and talents need to walk hand in hand with your charisma. Those who have figured out how to brand their unique combination of these factors are undoubtedly some of your favorite performers. Performance ability and charismatic performance are each incomplete without the other. As an actor or singer, you need to have both skill and charisma. The absence of either will prevent you from making your desired impact.

You know you have to learn and polish how to perform. Most of us believe that people are born with a natural knack for the performing arts, but we must consciously choose to pursue them if we want to be skilled. Similarly, you're born with charisma. You need to discover and develop it if you want to benefit from it. Did you notice the similarity here? In both cases, you need to improve these elements consciously. These qualities can lie hidden, but you can find and polish them. You'll need to dig deep to find these attributes. You may have both talent and charm, but unless you discover and develop them, they will hold no value.

If charisma is considered a divine gift, then talent is no different. Talent must be developed. Like charisma, it needs to be regularly practiced. You must practice achieving perfection in your performance, and you need to hone your charismatic skills to garner attention. When you've practiced your craft, you'll command attention from your audiences. No one will be able to look away from you. If used in the right way, these elements can prove to be a catalyst for fame.

AN OBSERVATION ON DRIVE AND TENACITY

You may have noticed, as I have, that many charismatic celebrities had unhappy childhoods without the love and affection children need during their growing years. They were either abandoned or lost their parents early in their lives. They became despondent and had low self-esteem; they felt deprived, lost, and out of place in society.

Nonetheless, each of these people later connected to their inner selves. Some very likely wanted to shine by outclassing others. They developed an art to which they dedicated themselves. Their actual motivations may have been different in each case, but once they realized they were gifted, nothing could stop them from achieving their dreams. They found a companion in these art forms and took them on as challenges. They didn't stop until they reached the pinnacle of their careers to prove to themselves that they could be of use to society—to be winners.

A few people of this type include John Lennon, Marilyn Monroe, Charlie Chaplin, Pablo Picasso, and Paul Gauguin. Eminem is a successful rap artist who explicitly talks about his abusive childhood in his songs. Besides these artists, many others all across the world who had similar backgrounds have used their charisma in positive ways and achieved fame.

I now want to share legendary Hollywood photographer Harry Langdon, Jr.'s story with you. He exudes charisma, is a dynamic personality and has always overcome the adversity in his life. He has worked with charismatic legends, is one himself and his father was one as well. I am in awe of his strong spirituality, beliefs, and perseverance.

"They say when we are planning our journey back here on the Earth Plane, we decide who would make our best parents. Right or wrong, we can have no complaints," insists Harry. "My dad was a famous comedian who died when I was ten in 1944. My mother was a beautiful East Indian actress that waited till recently to pass-on. I learned very early that having a famous parent could be an impediment. I realized at almost the time he died; I was on my own now".

"People would ask, so your father was famous, what do you do?" Harry confides. "That motivated me to make something of myself. I did art, oil painting and carpentry. I became a journeyman carpenter at 17. I had a Ham Radio station at 14. Then my mother bought photographic darkroom paraphernalia and that was the thing I needed to engage myself away from teenage mischief."

"I was so occupied with all these hobbies and work, that my mind could not imagine going out on a date. Plus, I was very shy and introverted, so again my mother enrolled me in an

Arthur Murray dance school. At the age of 18, I was transformed, and I became a gold medal champion at 19. I could now say I had accomplished something and made my contribution. But I always had my photography hobby, which gradually overtook my dancing adventures. The bashful kid had turned into being a gigolo".

"I began to photograph women that I met out dancing, then those photos caught the attention of modeling agencies in Los Angeles. Then those models' photos caught the attention of famous actors and actresses including Ann Margret, Diana Ross Tom Jones, President Ronald Reagan, Halle Berry, Sophia Loren, Raquel Welch, Joan Rivers, Robin Williams and many more, well into the 1000s which now I have in my digital archives".

"In the movies they say 'Fade-Out and Fade in,'" quips Harry. "I have been married and divorced three times to very beautiful women. I have had and still have a beautiful home and very luxurious cars. But, after all those wonderful temporary experiences, I have had exceptional revelations that there is a higher spiritual level we are all longing for".

"We all are consciously or perhaps unconsciously journeying toward those goals. There is not enough room here to describe what epiphanies I have had, as they are very sacred. I can only say that everyone should stay tuned in to those moments of divine inspiration that can perhaps lead the lowest, fallen person to break out into a life of indescribable extreme happiness that I am enjoying now. It may mean giving up self-destructive habits," he concurs.

"A photographer is surrounded by very worldly temptations. I fell for them. But, as successful as I was, I could not look into a mirror and be proud of myself when I was indulging in alcohol or drugs. Our spirit is there for us to look at in the mirror," he declares. "Until I went clean I was not able to see a rather handsome person again that I could be proud of".

"To summarize, now I live a very simple life by myself, surrounded by the trappings of an advanced photographer which is very high-end computer apparatus," Harry reveals. "I seldom date. I have been there and done that. I earn a comfortable living on royalties and occasional photo sessions. I owe this peaceful existence to a trust in the Creator, and am following his or her guidance every minute of the day and night.

One hint, he adds, is to avoid any grudgeful baggage. "Forgiveness is the key. It has been written, if we forgive, we will be forgiven. That may mean to forgive us as well. Yes, I had chosen the perfect parents," Harry Langdon, Jr. concludes.

The challenge lies in handling things with a positive spirit and never giving up the fight. We all know of many superstars who tread the wrong path that led to self- destruction, including Amy Winehouse, Kurt Cobain, and Whitney Houston. Yet there are examples of those who transformed their sorry state through creativity, such as Eric Clapton or Robert Downey, Jr. Their creativity helped them to reach the top in a constructive way.

Performing artists must be capable of providing their audiences with powerful and captivating performances. A performance that arrests the attention is often remembered forever, which is a primary aim of a true artist. And isn't that what charisma is all about?

Chapter 10

Charisma and Leadership

Charismatic leaders reach their followers in a basic, emotional way to inspire, motivate, and guide them. Leadership is all about charisma (and vice versa). A leader has to have charismatic qualities; why else would a bunch of people listen to someone? That person has what it takes to be the face of a group. A successful authority figure is strong willed, has mental strength, is a good orator, can inspire people, and above all, can influence them. A true leader can unite a group under his or her leadership, encouraging people to work toward a common goal.

In fact, the success of leaders rests in their charismatic personalities. Leaders have to look at broader perspectives that go beyond their personal limits. Their efforts to help others be successful in their lives should be limitless too. What makes a leader effective is the ability to see what others can't. This means that they need to put their own needs aside to help others. Remember that a candle doesn't lose anything by lighting the flame of another candle.

Charisma and personality have proven to be an especially effective combo for attracting people. Self-determination and strong control over desires make leaders who they are. Great administrators such as Donald Trump successfully spin an amicable environment around people and make them comfortable whenever they can. This brings out the humane side of any individual, which in turn earns them loyalty.

Many people believe that leadership skills and charisma are qualities you are born with. Leadership can be an inborn trait, but like charisma, with time leadership skills can be learned. There should be no end to learning, and there's no other way to attain perfection.

The importance of charisma in a leader's life is substantial. A leader needs charisma to help them connect to people to present a magnetic personality that draws the masses. Leaders try to remain unique and make their group exceptional and distinct.

Charismatic leadership is all about integrating, influencing, and inspiring people. Leaders can unite a group of people with varied backgrounds under one aim and help them achieve it.

THIS KIND OF LEADERSHIP HAS THE FOLLOWING TRAITS:

Awareness. As a leader, you need to be clear about what you want to do. Awareness is crucial. You must know your strengths, values and weaknesses. You must also be aware of how other people perceive you and your ideas.

Reliability. A charismatic leader has to be dependable. Only then will people find them worthy of trust. A trustworthy leader first wins the confidence of people and then lives up to it.

Consistency. An effective leader has to be consistent. You should follow through when you say you are going to do something. This builds trust and establishes your reputation.

Sanguinity. A charismatic leader is a positive thinker. You need to keep your followers motivated and encourage them to support you and one another.

Creativity. Charisma can make a leader farsighted. Leaders have to consider the future and have a good idea of the outcomes of their decisions. They need to analyze situations and strategize before they make their decisions.

Determination. Leaders have to work under high pressure and need to keep things together for others. They have to be decisive and to keep the big picture in mind. They have to foresee the end results of their decisions and focus on how to get there.

Responsibility for consequences. You set your goals and make decisions. While we readily accept praise for good choices, we must also accept the responsibility for bad ones. We must live with the results of the choices we make, either way. Think through the pros and cons of a situation before you act.

Whenever you get the opportunity to be chosen as a leader, point out these qualities in yourself. Really good leadership, like charisma, is built around virtues.

Charismatic leadership can change the world and make a difference. In the pages of history, you can find many examples of leaders whose charisma influenced people in many ways.

Chapter 11

Love and Charisma

People often find themselves wondering whether love has something to do with charisma. How are love and the charisma factor related? Is there any relationship between the two elements, or is that seeming connection merely an illusion created by the human mind?

Consider the love you share with your mother, sister, best friend, or boyfriend. Do you share a bond that makes your heart feel light and stress free when you're together? Can you share most of your worries, sorrows, and tensions while feeling relaxed and good? If your answer is yes, then you can surely understand the gravity of the point I'm trying to make.

Look at the power of someone whose presence turns your tears into a beaming and gleaming smile. The sense of security you feel near your loved ones is one form of charisma.

Does the charisma factor exist in every relationship that's built on the basis of love, care, and affection? Or does it apply only in certain special relationships? Which is the most charismatic relationship in your life? Everyone is curious about the one whom he or she considers the darling of his or her life.

I've been in love a couple of times. I had an on again-off again passionate relationship with Hollywood glamour photographer Harry Langdon in the late eighties through the early nineties. We were inseparable. Both of us were strong- willed, good-humored and dynamic personalities. There was no doubt we were in love and that this love was charismatic. I look back on our years together fondly.

Breakups are difficult. I learned a lot from Harry spiritually, I really did. I learned a lot from him about charisma as well. We had a real soul connection, and I truly loved him. Our breakup was difficult, and it took hard work to discover and develop my inner strength again. I am pleased to say that I have been in a loving relationship with a the love of my life and a wonderful man, Larry Wohl, for 13 years now and our love is indeed charismatic. It takes work, but, if I can do it, so can you!

I can demonstrate the charisma of love using a variation of something I learned in method acting. Do you remember when you came across your first love? Remember the feeling of butterflies in your stomach? The expression on your face, the blushes, the glow, and all the blessings that reminded you of them throughout the day. Even after sleepless nights, they still lingered in your thoughts.

Sit back. Relax. Breathe in and breathe out. Now follow the steps one by one, letting yourself feel loose and free enough to feel the experiences naturally. Don't be nervous or try anything artificial that can prevent you from discovering honest results.

- Think of a day when you were truly sad. You felt heartbroken and tired.

- Close your eyes and try to capture the moment exactly as it happened, while also feeling the pain you went through. Now ask yourself whom you wanted by your side to give you a shoulder to cry on, console you, and make you feel better.
- Next, remind yourself of your first crush. Think of the daydreams you had. :-)
- Count the number of people you love the most on this earth and those that love you too. Don't miss a single person you want to be with forever.
- Now scroll through the virtual list of names and search for the name of the person you want to be by your side during your tough times.
- You've found the one who sprinkles the impeccable charm of love in your life and who matters most to you.

Love can heal wounded hearts, help you deal with your troubles, and help you achieve what you want to accomplish in your life. Love is charismatic, and it exists in every individual, assisting in making people charismatic.

Apart from the love between two partners, there are various other forms of love. We love our kids, our friends, our family members, and our pets. I loved my cat to the moon and back, and he gives me back so much love and comfort that I miss him intensely when I'm away from him. It's no wonder that pets help people live longer and more fulfilling lives.

Love is a form of energy that beams through the body of all beings in the form of their expressions, feelings for one another, and in their behavior. Love is a pure feeling that spreads charm and joy in an amazing manner. People who feel loved and cared for are charismatic and hold the charm of happiness. All the love you feel for your parents, your siblings, your pets, your friends, or your life partners creates superb and blessed experiences. To love and be loved serves you with a warmth, happiness, and confidence that can keep you going even in the toughest times.

Love is charismatic, and it isn't only me saying this. Artists, writers, singers, and filmmakers have tried to portray love in their artistic creations because love is the central element that builds and preserves the charisma factor in human beings. Examples of the magnificent connection between love and the charisma factor are accepted and appreciated by people from all over the world.

I have always loved the following quote, drawn from the letters of Swami Vivekananda: "All love is expansion; all selfishness is contraction. Love is therefore the only law of life. He who loves lives, he who is selfish is dying. Therefore, love for love's sake, because it is the only law of life, just as you breathe to live."

What's the relationship between sex and charisma? It has been observed that the bodies of both males and females can glow after lovemaking. People feel happier, more energetic, and healthier. Sex is a seamless stress buster, and can drive away all your worries and offer you complete relaxation. But sexual intercourse is nothing but mere sex if no love is involved in it.

People who have a healthy lovemaking process and who share a great bond of physical relations with their partner are comparatively healthier and more active. These are the people who get sounder sleep after making love with their partners, which makes them feel more refreshed when they wake up in the morning—a great start to the day.

Now you must be wondering what all these things have

to do with the charisma factor, and how the benefits of sex can help promote charisma. Your concern is justified as long as you see sex merely as a fun, pleasurable, physical activity that offers you short-term gratification. However, when you explore the deepest aspects of sex, when it becomes one of the finest sources of the creation of energy through human bodies, you find your doubts disappearing. Sexual energy is pure and powerful. It's more than what people normally understand it to be. Those who are able to understand and consider the process of lovemaking as something magnificent can gain from it at a different level.

The major issue with our modern age is that people are more interested in instant fun and don't believe in the idea of creating and holding the natural power of sex. The process of rejuvenation through sexual energy includes various techniques that were developed in ancient times and have been preserved and carried forward into the contemporary world. However, in the hustle and bustle of modern life, which is hectic and often too busy, it's tough to pay attention to the things that are most important to living an enchanted life.

Especially for enjoying a strong, healthy, and charismatic sexual life, it's very important to pay complete attention to your lifestyle, making yourself energetic enough to have a good time in bed. To have an energetic and thrilling sex life, you need to be healthy. A body that gets tired after a full day's work can hardly retain enough stamina to have enthusiastic sex. To build your level of stamina, you need to adopt some daily exercises and a healthy diet, which will also help you to fill your life with charismatic experiences that reflect love and affection.

I adhere to a vegan diet and have since childhood, and

although I do this because I refuse to eat animals or animal by-products, I feel that my health is much better because of it. I generally feel vibrant, peppy, and exuberant throughout the day. I'm also not feeding my body the karma of an innocent being that was tortured and miserable throughout his or her life and died a violent death so that I could have a meal.

One major tip for building special sexual charisma in your body is to believe in your inner strength to create a new life. The first thing you need to do is get away from all insecurities related to your looks, sex appeal, and other personality attributes. You need to know that you're special in your own way; there's no need to be jealous of anyone else. Jealousy is by no means charismatic. Just pay attention to yourself and learn to modify your own existence, fixing your faults if required. Dumping the desire to be someone else is very important.

Before opting for any particular spiritual or body technique to build strength and power for sex, you need to understand that sex is the perfect source of a magnificent energy that rests in every individual. Understand the power of sex before using it. Emphasize converting this energy for your own good and without using other people, which can lead you to a happier and better life.

Keep in mind that the power of sex can actually create a baby. At the time of sexual intercourse, a special energy is released from the bodies of both mates. This energy brings them to a higher level of strength and stamina at which beings become capable of creating a new life. It is equivalent to the energy of the creator of this planet and all life upon it.

The power of love and sex has been a topic of interest since the beginning of time and has been the subject of many artistic endeavors including paintings, books, and films. Filmmakers have attempted to portray the power of love since the silent films of more than a hundred years ago. They give their best shots at showcasing the eternal and charismatic love the characters in their films share, but few of them have really succeeded.

James Cameron made an Oscar-winning film featuring the beautiful Kate Winslet and the charismatic Leonardo DiCaprio: Titanic. It's an epic about the undying love two people can share. The film is loaded with the charisma factor. Every time I watch it, I find it fresh and still appreciate the theme music, the first kiss of Rose and Jack at the bow of the gigantic ship, their sensual lovemaking, and the tragic ending. I feel nearly the same as I did while watching this film for the first time. The love shared by these two protagonists is everlasting, charismatic, and beyond the boundaries of life and death. Some people might not find this film to their tastes, but they can't deny the intensity of the love being portrayed.

The film deals with the popular concept of soul mates: two people who were made for each other. Even people who don't believe in this concept can feel and understand the importance of love in human life, which shows the stronger connection between love and charisma. Both are inherent elements in human beings and need complete care and attention to develop.

There are, of course, various other films whose directors and screenwriters have tried their best to represent charismatic love. The Twilight saga depicts love between a vampire and a human. The romance in this film comes charismatically alive on-screen, even though some people might find it hard to connect with the odd story line.

Fantasies are alluring enough to keep audiences trapped in

their charm, which explains the importance given to every lover in romantic films, books, and songs. Even as far back as the works of the great Shakespeare, love has been established as a great feeling, and romantic tales have been charismatic enough to keep their charm alive over the centuries.

IS EVERY LOVE CHARISMATIC?

Do you feel like the love between you and your partner can create magic in your life, or does it already? Many people are confused about the charm and power of the love in their relationships. Relationships grow and become more magnificent when they're nurtured with care, understanding, and attention.

But sometimes relationships end, which can be hard to handle, especially when the people involved can't find or don't understand the reasons that they fell apart. Many issues can be resolved by paying careful attention to the bond you share with your partner. Showering it with complete care and love is very crucial to keeping it going. Relationships can be successful and satisfying for both partners if they're based on mutual trust, care, and understanding.

Love and charisma are interrelated. One can't exist without the other. Charisma can't survive for very long without love. Look at this with a logical mind and an eye for detail. If people don't like or love you, they won't be smitten by your charisma. Usually when you attempt to fake it, people catch the deception and lose affection for you. You may be able to mislead them in the beginning, but sooner or later, people discover the truth. The steps below will guide you in attaining love and charisma the right way.

1. Learn to love yourself. While love can transcend all boundaries and be a powerful weapon in proving your points and convincing the multitudes, you need to start by loving yourself. You need to love yourself in order to spread love. This self-love will help you to be more focused and dedicated in your mission of preaching love. Love is a language the whole world comprehends. When you've learned how to love yourself, you'll be able to preach the tenets of love to others without a doubt in your heart. Moreover, people who can love themselves can make a difference by teaching others about love in a charismatic way.
2. Keep smiling. Love without a smiling heart can't be sustained. There has to be a twinkle somewhere in your face, even if you aren't in the mood. There is no need to explain that your smile should be warm and pleasant; it shouldn't look like a grimace or a smirk with nothing backing it up. It must be proportionate and natural, yet friendly. Charismatic personalities can have a lot to think about before they go out in public. The look they wear has to be pleasant yet intelligent. That's why you'll want to improve your personality before you begin flashing that killer smile of yours.
3. Be confident. Both love and charisma come to people who have confidence. Charismatic people are sure of what they want to do and are ready to face the consequences of their actions. This is the result of their confidence. If you're confident that your love will bring out a change in someone or some situation, pursuing that person or task will be worth it. Remember, if you can't help a person, do nothing to hurt them. This is part of the law of karma.

4. Be sincere. Never forget that old proverb, "Honesty is the best policy." If you really think that love should help carve out your charisma in a constructive way, it's best to be honest with yourself first and then with others. People who are true to themselves can win over others' hearts. When people can read the honesty in you, they're more apt to like you. There is no need to spell it out that sincerity begets true love.
5. Be sociable. Charismatic people are affable creatures, which makes others appreciate them more. There is no way you'll feel despised in your life because there will be many chances to fill your loneliness.

So, now you see that charisma and love are like two sides of the same coin. If you develop one, the other will accompany you like a loyal friend. You may wonder whether relationships that break weren't charismatic enough to last. Don't confuse love with relationships. Love is freedom, and relationships come with boundaries, although the two go hand in hand. Without love, no relationship can have a long life, but people sharing any bond of love should be aware of how to hold on to it. The charisma you hold within yourself in the form of internal love will help you deal with problems in relationships. Remember, love holds the power to heal wounds; hence, it can help you deal with the minor and major problems in any relationship. Free yet balanced love is the charisma factor. Have you got the quintessence of the charisma factor and love in you?

Chapter 12

Self-Discipline and Authenticity

The biggest difference between who you are authentically and becoming who you want to be is what you actually do. With self-discipline developed, the smallest decision can change the course of your life.

Let's say that one day you make the decision to quit smoking. You're fully aware of all the health issues related to it, you know that your family has always been against the habit, and you know all the pros and cons. But the next day, the day of execution, you fail to accomplish the task you have set up for yourself. Then you ask yourself why you failed to follow through with the decision. After a full analysis, an inner voice whispers, "You don't have the power or persistence to change this habit".

So many people are aware of the changes they need to make in their lives, but they don't know what keeps them from making them. How many times have you started to do something but quit after a short while? How many times have you said, "I wish I had stronger willpower?" How many times have you felt like a failure in your own eyes? Well, you aren't exceptional; we all experience this. We lack self-discipline.

WHAT IS SELF-DISCIPLINE?

Self-discipline is the ability to overcome your problems or to act regardless of your emotional state. Every one of us knows that we have a few habits we wish we could get rid of, such as laziness, excessive eating, smoking, procrastination, lack of assertiveness, or carelessness. To break these habits, one needs a certain degree of willpower. Self-discipline makes a great difference in everyone's life, bringing with it, inner strength, self-control, and power. Self- discipline is one of the key elements that can lead you to a successful life.

When you achieve self-discipline, you find the inner strength to guide yourself further in life. Your charisma will be enlightened, and you'll shine like a beautiful, twinkling star. The problems that self-discipline can solve are important, and while there are other ways to solve them, self-discipline is the best way. Self-discipline can empower you to overcome any addiction and help you to find your inner beauty. When you combine self-discipline, passion, planning, and your dreams, you come up with the charismatic personality that previously was hidden from you.

Self-discipline is a combination of willpower and determination, and it helps create charisma within you. It confers on us the ability to withstand difficulties and hardships, be they emotional, mental, or physical. It seems as if it gives us the ability to put a stop to our impulses because it helps us understand that we may gain something if we expend some effort and time. All of us have hidden desires we need to control in order to make our lives better: we will no longer be making rash decisions. Self-discipline gives us the power to control our minds and at the same time train them in a positive way to avoid looking for only instant gratification.

Imagine you'd like to lose some weight—let's say around fifteen pounds or so. Without the ability to restrain yourself, you will repeat the same mistakes you made that gained you those pounds in the first place. You need to hold yourself back and be determined to lose the weight. You need self-discipline. Apply it in your life. Once you are self- disciplined, you'll be able to teach others.

Self-discipline is the ability to abstain from making bad, impulsive decisions. You'll make decisions the right way and then stand by them without changing your mind. Self- discipline plays a significant role in achieving any goal.

It's a common belief that self-discipline is limiting and leads to a restrictive lifestyle. Instead, self-discipline is a giving quality, provided you trust it. It helps you make the right calls and choices and to have the strength to think; it leads you to success. It gives you the inner sight you've always wanted.

WHY SELF-DISCIPLINE IS IMPORTANT TO THE CHARISMA FACTOR

We need to rise to the occasion when we find ourselves in adverse situations. That's when you'll know that self- discipline is the best quality you could ever have developed. Such occasions demand that you remain focused so you can tackle any problems. If superficial things distract you, you may not be able to solve them in the best possible way. When you find yourself in adverse conditions, you need to gather all the courage you can and face up to things. If you're scared, self-discipline will come to your rescue, as your charisma factor is stimulated by it.

You can cultivate self-discipline. Inner strength gives you power to make decisions and efforts. People often feel too lethargic to do something they want to do, so they fail unless they're serious about changing to become stronger and better. When we adopt self-discipline, it's very easy to discover and sustain our charismatic characteristics. It's vital for learning and self-development. You will gradually get stronger, and your perception of life will change. With practice, self-discipline will become a habit that will lead you to growth and success.

Developing self-discipline will help you to:

- Mean what you say and keep your promises
- Avoid giving into momentary pleasure over long-term benefits
- Increase your output
- Be motivated to work hard
- Avoid becoming depressed
- Change and improve yourself
- Feel enthusiastic and energetic
- Do what you enjoy
- Believe in yourself
- Develop resilience
- Learn to be adaptive

But how can you generate the kind of self-discipline that has a long-term impact? Every time you decide to accomplish something, sooner or later you'll face your own resistance, which is the major hurdle in the path of success and growth. The first thing to do is to realize how important it is to develop self-discipline. Then work for it. Think about why you should create this habit within yourself. Think about all the benefits you will experience after you generate this trait that leads to miracles.

As you think about the miracles that come out of a disciplined life, be conscious of your own undisciplined side. You know that undisciplined behavior has an immediate impact on your life, but imagine the life you want to have in the long term. When you're aware of all the pros and cons of your own behavior, you'll be in a better place to plan your self-improvement. This will help you to sustain your charisma factor.

Make a wish list of all the things you want to achieve. I do this quite often. I did it with this book and with my animal welfare nonprofit organization Animal Ashram. Writing a list is helpful in generating visualization Your goals and aims, along with your priorities in life, go on the list. Visualize them. Your aspirations need to become your passion, and you'll do your best to accomplish the items on your list. Assert yourself. Manifest your dreams.

The charisma factor in you will help you to reach your dreams as you behave according to the decisions you've made, regardless of their hurdles and difficulties, procrastination, or the desire to give up. Just setting a goal isn't what's important; the work to get there is. What you are and what you do is the outcome of what you actually put in. Don't think that you can't change your behavior because it is possible. You need to inspire yourself by thinking of the power you'll gain. Your inner strength will help you overcome the biggest of problems.

The truth is, everything lies in the mind, and if you know how to control that, you can change your life. Your thinking can mature, gaining you inner strength and improving your powers of concentration. Master the art of being in charge of yourself, being more organized and focused. It will lead you toward spiritual growth and self-improvement.

BUILDING PILLARS OF SELF-DISCIPLINE

There are three pillars of self-discipline: acceptance, willpower, and hard work.

Once you accept your own flaws, you tend to be more accepting and aware of the need for self-discipline. When you discover your charisma, you polish it, and your spark generates positive vibes around you. But this charismatic factor is sustained only if you work continuously for it; gradually, it will become part of your personality. For that, you have to accept the changes you bring to yourself. Accept the way you are. Acceptance is the way to know yourself better and with confidence.

Strong willpower will help you to reach the place where you desire and deserve to be. Willpower is the only thing that keeps you motivated over the long haul. Strong willpower will help you persevere along your path. When you discover what you want to change or create in yourself, you continue on the track to accomplish your goal. But you'll find yourself resisting at times when your willpower isn't strong enough yet.

Once you decide to do something, work for it. Keep it as your ultimate goal. If you're overweight and decide to shed extra pounds, only your willpower will keep you motivated enough to reach your goal. Only a strong willpower will keep you on the right track to your dreams rather than give in to the voice in your head that wants to hold you back.

Self-discipline is like a muscle that needs to be trained, and the more you train it, the stronger you become. Everyone is born with different strengths and reaches different levels of self-discipline. For example, not everyone can develop the discipline of holding his or her breath underwater for a long time.

The basic method of building self-discipline is to face challenges. Get out of your comfort zone, but keep your goals realistic; there's no reason to set impossible goals. Be a doer. Doers are a rare species, and they believe in what they do. They don't give up halfway, and neither should you. Doers complete what they start; they set possible goals. The bottom line is, if you think it's not possible to change through positive thinking, you've created a self-fulfilling prophecy, and you'll probably never accomplish anything. The final pillar of self-discipline is hard work; it's necessary to success, and it always pays off. You have to work to get where you're going; mere thinking can't help you achieve your dreams.

The science around willpower is very compelling. In one of the most renowned studies, Dr. Walter Mischel and his colleagues at Stanford University in the 1970s, tested elementary school children. When first taken into the workroom children were told that they could eat one marshmallow right away or wait and eat two marshmallows in a few minutes. The treats were always visible to the children. If the child couldn't wait, they could ring a bell and the researcher would come back and give them the one marshmallow, but they wouldn't get the second one. They followed these children for years and demonstrated that the kids who had more self-control and could delay their gratification in that experiment became generally more successful and healthier across the lifespan than their more impulsive friends. They were able to perform better at school and resist such negative habits and traits such as drug use, alcoholism and obesity.

Even more enlightening is the recent neuroscience research that shows that actual physical changes in the structure of the brain occur when people act less impulsively. In other words, the brain changes when you practice self-discipline, specifically the frontal lobe, which is the key decision-making and executive function part of the brain, grows stronger and thicker, while the emotional areas, the fight or flight center of the brain called the amygdala becomes a little weaker and appears to shrink.

Interestingly the same pattern of brain change occurs when people meditate and/or practice virtues like compassion and forgiveness. The key part of this science of brain change is that such structural changes only occur when you behave differently. You brain doesn't change just by thinking, you need to act differently.

Simply look at where you are now and aim to get better as you go forward. You won't do justice to yourself if you ask others to do what you should do for yourself. Learn how to strike the correct balance in order to reach your destination.

People with self-discipline rarely give up. They definitely place work before pleasure. After completing a day's work, they relax without feeling guilty. The charisma factor in you can be stimulated and sustained once you've cultivated self- discipline. Imagine the life that has no direction and no goal to accomplish. Life can only be delightful once you treat yourself in a special way and never give up.

Chapter 13

Tools and Techniques for Developing Charisma

As we've discovered, charisma can be worked on and developed with practice. You already know that you must connect with yourself to become a truly charismatic person. You must overcome any negative thoughts so that your positive energy emerges. Knowing yourself and discovering your purpose in life was your very first step. Accept your talents as the gift from the Almighty that they are, allow them to motivate you, acknowledge your strengths (and work on your weaknesses so you can turn them into strengths). Have faith in and respect yourself and have gratitude for the people who have contributed to your life. Only then can you move on to the next steps in building your charismatic personality.

DEVELOPING YOUR CHARISMA QUOTIENT

If you really want to develop charisma, you need to give it some time. Be patient; it takes a while for your inner glow to work its way outward.

This is how you can perfect the charisma quotient in yourself:

Body language. Standing straight will exude a positive energy that won't look forced but relaxed.

Positive attitude. Keep a positive attitude. It will help you in all possible ways, and people will notice. And if you have a smile on your face as well, you'll be well on your way to using your charisma factor to charm others.

Work on your style. Style includes all kinds of things. Wear smart clothes and avoid loose clothing that makes you look like you're wearing a sack. Create a style of speech that people might one day try to copy, to your delight. Charisma is about more than just looking good and stylish, but the whole package you offer to others is important.

Avoid pretense. It's imperative that you be straight with people. You need to be frank and say things clearly.

Take your time. Slow down while speaking, acting, working, and thinking. Don't be in a hurry to save the world. First think, then talk, and after that, act.

Be flexible. Don't be obstinate about anything, and always be open to change, even if you don't like it right away. There may be options you can choose from when things aren't to your liking, but you'll need to be able to bend when things change.

So, you see, there are tricks to developing your charisma, but remember to practice if you aim to master these techniques.

Ordained Swami Priest Robin Cofer says you need to find your bliss and follow it. Specialize in your bliss. "It will show all over your face and will be bursting forth from you. People will want to know your secret. Keep asking yourself, 'What do I love, what do I love?' Figure out what your passion is and pursue it".

Find out what is new in people's lives by genuinely inquiring about them. Be generous and nurturing with your energy and be sincere.

Throughout this journey, we have discussed many aspects of charisma, but some people may be wondering what steps to take during the transition phase. Here are a few powerful tips that anyone can use to make themselves more likable, believable, and, ultimately, more charismatic. Practice them regularly, and gradually they will simply become part of your personality.

Calm down. The first and foremost thing is to relax and collect yourself. Charisma is all about channeling your energy toward whomever you meet. If you channel anxiety and stress, people will obviously be repelled. You have to be calm and relaxed enough so that when you meet people, they will feel relaxed and be attracted to your calmness. You have to understand that many people will be nervous and stressed, so take a deep breath, believe in yourself, and move forward.

Be enthusiastic. When you're passionate and enthusiastic, you connect with people more strongly and can convey emotions with ease. Your passion is reflected in your work, words, and deeds. When you're enthusiastic, people who meet you will feel your high spirits. One thing that usually strikes us about successful entrepreneurs is their degree of enthusiasm, which is appealing and connects with the masses. That's the reason many of them are charismatic leaders and impressive personalities.

Be confident. Charisma isn't only about being confident, but confidence always makes you more charismatic. When you're confident, people will be more at ease with you and are more likely to trust you. Your confidence will boost their energy level. It's commonly suggested that even if you aren't feeling confident, you should pretend to be because real confidence is something that comes with knowledge and practice.

Carry yourself correctly. It's said that you speak even before you open your mouth. You convey a silent message by the way you carry yourself. Project yourself as a charismatic personality: physically, emotionally, and intellectually. I won't suggest that your first impression is your last impression, but I will say that your first impression is long lasting. When you're at ease, you tend to carry yourself better and project more strongly.

Speak well. You may have a terrific idea, but no one will know about it until and unless you can articulate it. You have to speak well. Think before you speak and try to make every word count. Think about how you're going to phrase things before you start talking. If you omit all the fluff from your daily communications, your words will be more sensible and reasonable. People will love to listen to you.

Always remember that if you don't have anything important to say, it's better to be quiet. In fact, limiting your words will make people more interested in what you say. Your silence will speak louder than your words. When you practice talking correctly, the right words will come to you more often. Also, speak with conviction. The way you say something is as important as what you say.

Make your presence felt. If your presence is strong, people will be more likely to feel your absence. Being present means having moment-to- moment awareness of what is happening around you and not letting your thoughts wander or being stuck in your own thoughts. If you become distracted in the middle of a conversation, your eyes will glaze over, and your facial expressions and body language will change. Others will easily notice that you are lacking good presence of mind and that you are only present physically.

Treat people as they want to be treated. This doesn't mean you have to please everyone, but when you make each person you meet feel important; they will feel good about themselves, and that will lead to a change in their perception of you. Treat them as if they're very important and their presence is remarkable. Gradually, people will be drawn to you, and they'll begin to hold a high opinion of you. Simple things, like remembering people's names to use every time you speak to them, when complimenting them, greeting them genuinely, smiling, empathizing, accepting compliments graciously, listening patiently and responding accordingly, making continuous eye contact, nodding and shaking hands firmly all make people feel more connected to you.

Get in touch with your emotions. Charismatic people feel their emotions strongly, which is why they are able to connect with other people's emotions. In many societies, expression of emotions isn't desirable, but you shouldn't be afraid to feel your own emotions. Instead of suppressing your emotions, control the way you express them.

Develop a warm personality. It is well known that a friendly personality attracts people and makes you charismatic, but a warm personality makes others feel even better. You can create a warm personality by connecting with people the best you can. Work to enjoy the company of others and appreciate them for what they are. If you force this quality, people will notice. Be genuine and honest with yourself and others. When you are stubborn and stuck on something, no one who meets you will want to listen to you. Open your arms, welcome them, and show the refreshing and warm personality in you. Welcome each new thing and a person in your life with the same conviction, as you want to be welcomed in your life.

Be visionary. Visionary ideas can change lives. People admire those who think for themselves as well as of others. One example of communicating a great vision came from the very famous entrepreneur Steve Jobs. To bring the then CEO of Pepsi, John Sculley, on board at Apple, he asked, "Do you want to sell sugar water the rest of your life? Or do you want to come with me and change the world?" What other option was open to Sculley except to take up the challenge?

Be positive. Spread happiness around you. Have fun. Charismatic people are always fun to be around. Be happy inside and carry it along with you. Don't regret anything you've done in the past. Learn a lesson from any regrets. Play; be creative, engage in a hobby or whatever else makes you happy. Always keep a gentle smile on your face; this will welcome the positive energies around you.

"If you feed a negative thought it will grow in strength. A moment of anger may produce the thought, 'I hate my husband.' The more attention and energy you give this thought, the more power it has over you. The next thing you know, you are divorced. Don't feed the thought. Immediately use an affirmation, i.e., 'every day in every way, our relationship is healing; I am learning how to forgive, how to love, how to heal", says Cofer.

Come out of your comfort zone. To be exceptional, to be charismatic, to be adorable and noticeable, you have to have something different and unique about you. People only do what they think they can do. Intentionally put yourself in uncomfortable situations so you can come up with ways to deal with the discomfort more effectively and efficiently. Anyone can perform well within his or her comfort zones; the champion is he or she who can sail the ship against the wind. Challenge yourself. Kick a bad habit. Find a new hobby. Volunteer. Take a class about something that interests you. Journal every day. Meditate. Spend time getting to know your authentic self. This will prepare you for any adversity you may face. . It will also help make people want to follow you; they'll admire you for your resilient personality.

Don't compare yourself to others. Everyone has their own reasons for doing what they do. It is human nature to compare ourselves to others. If it's done in a healthy way—to find motivation—it can be good, to a point. But when you criticize yourself in comparisons, it's a problem. The Almighty has given potential and strength to each of us. Don't imitate others blindly. Don't ever criticize yourself for not being someone else. Keep your blinders on. If you're comparing yourself, it clearly means you think someone else is superior to you. If you don't believe in your own power, no one else will. Trust yourself and believe that you were destined to accomplish great things. Comparing not only affects your own personality, it may also affect how others perceive you.

Listen. Listen to what your heart and mind say and act accordingly. After you've listened to yourself, you should get into the habit of listening to others. You can become an excellent listener by listening deliberately, pausing, and questioning. When you listen to people carefully, you'll give them the feeling you're with them completely. Patient listening is key to opening a line of communication that makes others feel special. Most of us wait for others to finish speaking completely to show they've been listening carefully and then take their turn to speak. However, asking questions gives people the feeling you've been totally involved in the conversation. Sometimes all people really want is to have someone listen patiently, and then their problem is half solved.

Know that looks don't matter. To be charismatic, you don't have to be the most attractive person in the room. Rather, you need to be magnetic. Good looks bring an added advantage, but they aren't a requirement for being charismatic. There's an endless list of people who aren't particularly attractive but are exceptionally charming and have such a sparkling personality that millions want to follow them. Charisma is beyond looks and appearances. It comes from within and reflects outward. Be the most attractive person from your heart, and you'll stand out in a crowd.

Know your power. Know your own power and explore it. A full charismatic package is the magic combination of your power and the warmth of your personality. Physical strength isn't true power; power comes from within. Kindness is the power of Princess

Diana and Melania Trump. , while intelligence is the power of Steve Jobs and Mike Pompeo. These charismatic personalities may not be physically powerful, but their personas are so strong that millions of people try to be like them. When you increase the level of your power, your level of charisma also increases.

The potential to be charismatic is within you; developing it is an art. All the small tips in this chapter can help you to be more charismatic, but charisma comes from within and should never be forced. Practicing these simple actions will help you realize that becoming charismatic isn't tough; it relies mainly on simple, small things. Maybe you won't follow all the tips, but at least try most of them. Nobody's perfect. You will have to decide where you want to stand and what your priorities and preferences are.

We can all apply these elements of charisma to our personal lives, jobs, and social situations—in any setting where the ability to attract others can be beneficial. The best thing about charisma is that you can become more powerful without making others less so because charismatic power is personal rather than positional power. You aren't competing for power with anyone; it's inside you. To be more powerful, just polish it.

Identify the major personality traits of other charismatic personalities and adopt them into your behavior. Develop and identify your core personality. You should also understand the difference between being charismatic and pleasing people. Charismatic people don't pay much attention to what people think about them. They enjoy being charismatic and charming on their own.

Developing Charisma 1: The Magic of Learning and Change

If you read many of the self-help experts and behavior change specialists, they will often tell you—in no uncertain terms—that trying to change your behavior can be a real pain, literally and metaphorically. When people try to change their diets, for example, they often have some success at first but sooner or later (typically sooner) the dieter goes back to her old ways.

There's a lot of research on this because lifestyle change is a key not just to a healthier life but a more successful and meaningful one. However, change can be hard and I have found some depressing information that suggests that people trying to change any behavior—cutting back on drugs (legal or otherwise), trying to quit drinking, or change eating patterns—all have relatively low rates of success.

However, before you get too discouraged, there is something different about charisma. Learning how to become charismatic is rarely painful, and often joyful. Learning how to become charismatic is a thrill, not a deprivation. Learning how to become charismatic is intrinsically rewarding in a way that avoiding ice cream, chocolate and your favorite desserts isn't. There is no deprivation in becoming charismatic.

The problem with changing behaviors like eating, smoking and drinking, is that there is an initial period of deprivation and difficulty before you start seeing the results of your efforts. That's not the case with learning to be charismatic. The journey is often joyous and rewarding from the very beginning. As your power, purpose and potential grow, there is not just a behavioral change but a spiritual one that echoes through your very soul.

Now, just because learning to become charismatic is potentially a wonderful journey, doesn't mean that the principles of learning and behavior change do not apply. Far from it. They are very important. So, let me show how to approach the process of making yourself more charismatic.

I reached out to friend of mine who as an expert in this field and he showed me some tools and resources that are used by people specializing in helping people learn and change.

The first thing he showed me was something called *The Stages of Change Model.* This was devised in the eighties by two psychologists working in the addiction field and has since become used in many different specialties. The original idea came from the experience that many therapists and others had while trying to help addicts and alcoholics. Many of these professionals were talking to the addict assuming that he or she had already decided to accept treatment when that was often not the case. It was recognized that you had to meet the addict where he or she was at, not where you thought they were. The model helped identify where anyone was at in the process of change and learning, and allowed professionals to adapt their communication accordingly.

There are five stages in this model:

Precontemplation. In this phase a person isn't even aware of the need or desire to change specific habits. This could be, for example, a smoker who isn't in the least interested in quitting his habit, or you the reader who up to this point had never considered trying to make yourself more charismatic.

Contemplation. This is the stage when a person is consciously aware that change might be needed or desired. This is the "I'm thinking about it" stage.

Preparation. This is when the person has accepted that she/he wants to change and begins the process for planning how that will happen.

Action. This is the stage where people take action to bring about the desired changes.

Maintenance. This is the critical stage of continuing what you started. As I mentioned above, it's very common for people to start something, like a new diet, but soon they are out of the action phase and typically back to contemplation as in "I'm not sure I want to keep doing this," or even worse, "I don't think I can do this."

It is important to note that people move in and out of these stages all the time. It would be awesome if we all moved smoothly through these stages and were able to change our behaviors so easily. Unfortunately, it generally doesn't happen as easily as that. But WAIT! We're talking about charisma.

The only reason for any precontemplation as far as charisma

is concerned is that the person hasn't realized that she can acquire it. Once you understand that you can learn to be charismatic, why would you need to think about it? Why would you even have to consider whether you wanted something that made you more powerful, successful, fulfilled, attractive and inspirational? Yes, you may have some reservations about whether you can actually do it, but surely the goal of leading a more purposeful and influential life requires little thought? And if it does, you need to start being more charismatic right now.

Self-belief is actually a characteristic of charisma. So, the very first step on your charisma journey is to accept that you can become charismatic.

Put all doubt aside. Make the commitment to yourself. You are going to do this. You are not going to try it, you're going to do it.

As Yoda says, "Do or do not, there is no try."

Now the third stage of Preparation is important. Having made the commitment to become more charismatic, it is helpful to plan the best ways of achieving your goal.

Preparation guidelines come from asking questions that apply to any change or learning process.

How am I going to stay focused on learning to be charismatic? What do I have to do in order to develop charisma?

How will I ensure that I am doing—and keep doing—what I need to do?

Those are three critical questions that focus on the core issue of change, the 3 M's: Motivation, Methods and Maintenance.

MOTIVATION

Even the most charismatic people have times when their energy is low or are swamped with stressors, or are in environments that aren't conducive to the behaviors they are trying to develop or maintain. Motivation can be like the tide, washing in and out of your mind-body and leading you to swim in the high tide of excitement or flounder in the receding force of nature.

What can help overcome these waves of energy is COMMITMENT. You need to be committed, no matter what. No matter what else is happening, you are committed.

There may be times when you have to change your plans, but this is adaptation not a loss of motivation or a reduction in your commitment. Charismatic people are adaptive and resilient. They don't quit, they just find a different way to make it work. You might need to turn your power down occasionally, but you never turn it off.

There are several simple ways to drill your charisma commitment into your consciousness.

Create a mantra or a phrase that captures your charisma commitment. For example, you might write down on sticky notes "Charisma is a Charm." (You might have noted that 'is a Charm' is an anagram of Charisma.) Or simply, "I Am Charismatic" or "Fulfilment and Joy through Charisma." Then post the sticky notes all over your environment so you can't escape them. Write the phrase or mantra down at the beginning of every day.

Make associations between your charisma commitment and everyday behaviors. For example, associate your car keys with your commitment. Your commitment is key. Every time you start the car, remind yourself that you're on the next part of your journey, not just to the grocery store or work but to fulfilment, inspiration and purpose. Or associate taking a shower with the power of charisma. Water is a force of nature that cleanses and heals, like charisma. Rhymes help—so consider 'the Power of the Shower.' Or associate coffee with charisma—both are energizing.

Visualization is a key part of motivation. Visualization is practice. Lots of scientific studies have shown that when you imagine yourself doing an action, it's almost as effective as actually physically doing it, in terms of learning. It's why many professionals, from sports stars to entrepreneurs, visualize themselves achieving their goals. Not only does seeing yourself achieve a goal and reinforce your motivation, but it is also actual practice.

Visualization is a great way to breach the gap between where you are now and where you want to be. For example, it would be great if you were to give an inspiring speech to your co-workers. Now that might not be possible right now, because the opportunity isn't there. However, visualizing yourself giving that speech, enables you to practice it now.

Visualization is therefore a great way to rehearse several charismatic behaviors without necessarily being in the situation to do them in "real life." In addition, when you mentally rehearse charismatic behaviors, your emotional response will give you clues as to how your behavior might need to be changed or upgraded. For example, as you visualize going to the podium to make your speech you might feel apprehensive or nervous, something that needs to be addressed in real life, through visualization.

Remember, too, that charisma is about appearance. So, visualization is important in that it provides that critical visual perspective to your behavior.

METHODS

In the sections that follow, I will be giving specific tools about how to develop the different aspect of charisma: Communication, Appearance, Mindset, Emotional Intelligence, Lifestyle and Virtues. In these sections, I will outline what you need to develop and how to do that.

Learning is a very individual process. Each person starts with their own set of skills, talents, preferences and experience. While in the following chapters I give the specifics of what to do to develop charisma, feel free to use your own talents and interests to adapt these tools to your own personal situation.

MAINTENANCE

As I mentioned earlier, charismatic people always follow through on what is important to them, even under the most difficult circumstances—especially the most difficult circumstances. They don't quit. They keep doing what they need to do to continue to develop and improve.

The continued practice of the key charismatic behaviors is important as you are developing charisma, and once you have it developed. Here are some tools that help you do that.

1. Keep a record of your behavior. Each week, at least, review how well you did with your charismatic development. Keep

a journal and write down your experiences. What did you learn? How could you have handled it differently? For example, say you go to a social event. Did people respond to you the way you hoped? If so, why was that? If not, why was that? Look at the big picture, as well as the small one. How are you doing compared to say, three months ago?

2. Get support, ideally from someone who is charismatic or is trying to develop it. The values of support include accountability, feedback, tools, motivation, and inspiration. Practice with each other or in a small group.
3. Celebrate your successes. Reinforcement is an important part of learning, so give yourself credit when you get it right.

These general resources are important for overall learning and behavior change. And there will be natural forces that will drive you forward. The power you feel when you can communicate effectively and see how others respond to you. The joy you feel when others revel in the beauty of your soul that you can now express so clearly to yourself and others. The satisfaction you naturally derive from inspiring others. All of these are natural, incredibly powerful reinforcers that will be the reminders and an assertion that you are on the right path.

Developing Charisma 2: Communication

Human beings are social animals. We were made to connect with each other to provide support, love, care, and inspiration. We are made to be interdependent, in some obvious and some not-so-obvious ways. Whichever way you look at it, communication is a critical and powerful tool that we are all given and have the ability, if not the opportunity, to develop.

We have language, and words can be incredibly powerful. We also have non-verbal communication, the ability to perceive someone's intentions through gestures, expressions and body language. I recently discovered a misunderstanding that I have had for a long time about non- verbal communication.

I read somewhere a long time ago, that 93% of all communication is non-verbal. This is still widely accepted and preached by many people. Being an actress that made perfect sense to me, because I didn't just have to learn the words in the script but the way I would present them non- verbally. However, I have since discovered that widely quoted statistic is misleading. Originating in a psychology study in the 1960s, the research was conducted by psychologist Albert Mehrabian.

In that study, the experimenter said a very few words that were contradictory to the emotions he was showing. Most subjects said that in this situation, non-verbal cues were far more important than the very few (and seemingly contradictory) words that were spoken. However, most of the time, people speak more words and typically they are not contradictory to their non-verbal behaviors. Where they are, the non-verbal behaviors are trusted as more reliable than contradictory words.

So, words do matter, as do the non-verbal behaviors that accompany them. The words and the non-verbal behaviors need to complement each other if you want to be a good communicator.

The non-verbal behaviors that matter include expressions, gestures. movements, and posture.

I also learned something really cool about these behaviors. When we see someone performing an action, like punching the air in triumph, there are parts of our brain that almost copy those same actions. We have circuits in our brain that copy the behavior we see. These circuits don't actually involve the full movement of, for example, punching the air in triumph, but activate many of the small brain sub- programs involved in that action. This is the basis of empathy and compassion. We start to copy the behavior that we see and the emotions that are consistent with that behavior begin to rise within us.

Just think about what that really means. Our consciousness and mind react almost before we realize it. We are programmed to be able to put ourselves automatically into other people's situations—if they represent them correctly. The actor that delivers that amazing speech is reaching into our subconscious and influencing our thoughts and emotions.

Think about how amazingly powerful that is! With the right words and actions, you can automatically start a cascade of brain activity that changes the listener's emotional state.

When you have mastered the ability to use words and non-verbal actions to this level, you have immense power.

It's tempting to say that words are the ideas and the non-verbal behavior is the emotion that accompanies the message. When both are consistent and strong, the message is incredibly powerful.

However, words can be more powerful than most of us imagine. As you might expect, being an actress, I am very interested in this topic and have researched and practiced some skills.

Words are processed in different parts of the brain depending on their meaning. For example, the word "passed" is processed in different brain areas depending on the different meanings it has in the following sentences.

"I passed my exam".
"I passed the house where I grew up".
"I passed up the opportunity".

In addition, words can elicit images and emotions. Consider:

"Your example can affect your workforce".
"You can inspire your workforce".
"You have the power to transform your workforce with a tsunami of support and inspiration".

See the difference? *Feel* the difference?

There has been some psychological research that shows how words and ideas are framed influences perception. In one study on memory, how a photo was described changed the subject's memory as well as perception.

Subjects were shown the photo of an auto accident. Subsequently, they were asked to recall whether there was any broken glass in the road in the photo. Subjects who were told the cars "smashed" into each other were much more likely to recall broken glass in the photo than those who were told that the cars "hit" each other. In reality, there was no broken glass in the photo.

The use of imagery and metaphors is thus a very powerful tool for the charismatic communicator. It is a way of shaping the perception of the listener. Using powerful and spectacular images, and thus influencing the mind of the listener, is a way of creating the desired emotions. For example, using the Himalayas or Mount Everest as a metaphor, will almost inevitably fill listeners 'minds with spectacular images of beauty, challenge and achievement.

Another communication tool that is powerful when used appropriately is the use of the rhetorical question.

In most communication you are trying to get someone to identify with your sentiments, and point of view. The least effective way of doing this is ramming something down their throat and forcing them to agree with you. The secret to effective communication is getting the person to own the idea themselves. Rhetorical questions allow you to frame how your audience thinks about the problem.

I have a therapist friend. When someone comes to him to quit smoking, he starts by asking: "Why the heck do you want to quit?"

Why? Because he suspects that everyone else, including other health professionals, will have given the smoker their reasons why he should quit. It is far better to present that question in a way that allows the smoker to tell the truth, e.g. I'm ambivalent about quitting. In short, the onus is on the smoker to reach his own conclusions, not ones thrust on him by well-meaning people who don't understand effective communication. When people reach their own conclusions, they are much more likely to own the idea.

Now framing is how the media—and everyone else—tries to influence the listener's reaction.

I'm sure you can tell the difference between these headlines.

"Stock Prices Slump as Economy Crashes"

"Investors Cautious as Business Wavers"

Framing also comes into play by asking questions.

Framing questions properly highlights the issues you are trying to get across.

By framing the following sentence differently, it can have two different meanings.

"Ask not what your country can do for you, ask what you can do for your country," said John F. Kennedy, as he emphasized the need for more cooperation rather than selfish dependency.

It also uses another powerful communication technique which is contrast. Contrast means to vary greatly and in sentences it is used to show contrasting ideas. An example would be, "New York City was bustling with energy before COVID-19, but is now like a ghost town."

The world is very complex but reducing it to a simple binary, either/or question makes the choices much clearer. Note that if you were talking to a different audience and wanted to make the reverse point about the responsibility of government, you could use exactly the same words to the same effect.

"Ask not what you can do for your country, but what your country can do for you."

Analogies are also valuable tools for the charismatic communicator. Comparing a situation to an everyday occurrence arouses the listener's emotional response. The idea connects with the listener's experience.

So, for example, if you wanted to address how fake news can have a damaging effect on your organization you might say something like this: "False information about us is like a virus. It gets transmitted very easily, and if too many people catch it and think this is true, we will all soon be on a ventilator".

Stories are also another powerful way to connect to the listeners by transporting them into a situation where their emotional response can lead them to your message. For example, if you were trying to encourage resilience during a difficult time you might tell a story like this.

"I know someone who was held as a prisoner-of-war in Vietnam. He was beaten badly and he was starved but he never gave up. He was held in solitary confinement for months and was tortured, but he never gave up. He saw his fellow prisoners die in squalor, but he never gave up. He was left for hours in the burning sun but he never gave up. He was crushed, humiliated but the harder it got, the more determined he was. He survived and then thrived. There's nothing like surviving the ultimate ordeal and winning".

And it would help if you can truthfully add, "That man was me." Or my father. But definitely not my 'dad.' The word 'dad' reduces the man to mere ordinary mortality but the word "father" has a sense of power and presence, like God Himself.

In summary, your charismatic communication should involve connecting with your audience by comparing the situation to similar experiences and contrasting the ideas to make it clearer what is at stake.

Another tactic is providing a list of things that need to be done. Ideally this shouldn't be too long otherwise people won't remember it and you also have the risk of losing them. Some say a list of three is ideal: not too short, not too long. A list gives the idea that once those three things have been achieved, the problem will be solved. It makes it sound doable.

"All we have to do to beat this virus is increase testing, protect the vulnerable, and ensure our health system can continue to cope with the demand".

Now the astute reader will realize that, while three main goals are presented, there are many sub-goals that need to be met. But the list simplifies the issue and makes it seem manageable.

Another charismatic communication tactic is to relate the message to values and its moral foundations. This is done to state the real meaning and purpose of the message and actions.

For example, during the coronavirus pandemic, one of the biggest concerns was whether hospitals could cope with an extreme influx of cases. One way of charismatically presenting that problem would be to reduce it to its core moral foundation.

You can achieve that by phrasing a sentence like this:

"It's not fair or reasonable to ask doctors to make the decision as to who should live and who should be left to die".

Passion and commitment can also be communicated by setting high goals. Setting high goals may not always be realistic, but it sounds powerful and can be inspirational.

"Our plans and goals are nothing less than making us the

leading company, not just here in America, or just North America or even in Europe, but across the entire world!"

To summarize, the charismatic verbal communication tactics we have discussed here are using imagery and metaphors, framing, contrast, analogies, stories, lists and relating messages to morals and values.

CHARISMATIC NON-VERBAL COMMUNICATION

Verbal strategies are great, but they won't be very effective if they are not accompanied by the appropriate tone of voice, gestures and posture.

Imagine any of the quotes mentioned above being delivered in a monotone! Or with blank facial expression or slumped in a chair.

If you're delivering a powerful message, your tone needs to reflect that power. Loud, deliberate with emphasis in the right places. So, in the quote above about becoming the leading company in the world, the emphasis needs to be on "the entire world". Each of those last three words read slowly and loudly for emphasis, The. Entire. World.

Now, of course, your body language needs to reflect the power of the message. Perhaps as you deliver the end of this message, your fists are clenched, or your arms opened wide in a defiant gesture of success. There's more on non- verbal influencers in the chapter on appearance,

The setting in which the message is delivered adds to the power of the message. You can give this speech at a Board meeting in front of a few people, or at a gathering of employees. However, the speech is more appropriate for a large gathering.

In a smaller, more intimate setting you might take a different approach, speaking more directly to the people to develop a more personally meaningful message. Have you ever wondered why the final scene in so many movies take place in more public places rather than the intimacy of a small room?

A couple finally declaring their love for each other is much more powerful when done in public. There's something more committed about it. It seems more real and powerful if hundreds of people are observing it.

Finally, the tools of charismatic communication apply to self-talk as well. You are the one who listens to yourself more than anyone else. How do you frame your thoughts? What would happen if you framed your ideas and thoughts in the inspirational ways described in this section?

The tools outlined here are valuable guides to learning and developing charismatic communication, without which it is difficult to be truly charismatic.

Developing Charisma 3: Mindset

The charismatic person has the right mindset for success. They have to think effectively, be open-minded, be creative, and not be fixated on opinions and beliefs.

A few years ago, Stanford University psychologist Carol Dweck wrote a great book, *Mindset: The New Psychology of Success*. In it, she outlined the reasons why the right mindset was so important for success. She describes two fundamental types of mindset.

The first is called the *Fixed Mindset*. In this state the person is close-minded and very fixed in their views. They never are prepared to change their mind nor even consider alternative opinions and ideas. As a result, they are very rigid and not creative at all. Moreover, not only do they see the world that way, more importantly, they see themselves that way. They see their talents as fixed and limited with little possibility of improvement.

The second is called the *Growth Mindset*. The opposite of the fixed mindset, the person with this attribute is not only willing to learn and expand their consciousness, people with a growth mindset can see the endless possibilities for improvement and development of their talents.

Those with a growth mindset are much more likely to be successful in life. They are constantly evolving and looking ways to advance their skills and talents. Because life is a constant challenge, those with a growth mindset develop a resilient and adaptive approach that helps them through the inevitable obstacles.

People who are adaptive and resilient are inspirational. They have multiple stories of how they overcame countless obstacles, some of which seemed insurmountable. We all can relate to facing unseen challenges and have an instinctive admiration for those who can rise to the challenge and win. We have admiration for the person who simply refuses to give up because we know how difficult it is to persevere in the face of overwhelmingly unfavorable odds. Success is one thing, but success earned through perseverance and resilience against tough odds, is truly inspirational.

The charismatic person, therefore, isn't someone who has easily succeeded at everything they have ever tried. They are not the person who floats through life successfully fulfilling their dreams without encountering obstacles, which is not only a test of credibility but also potentially an object of scorn rather than praise.

Admitting flaws and failures but showing how resilience and adaptation moved you from the shame and humiliation of those lows to the grace of your successes, inspires people. It makes them see you as a real person. It makes you seem like the hero of your story, and maybe theirs.

The growth mindset is therefore not only critical for success, but is an essential part of helping others see you as creative, resilient and adaptive.

As Dweck's work was embraced, especially by educators, it naturally got a bit distorted. It became an all-or-nothing, binary proposition. Either you had a growth mindset, or a fixed mindset. Obviously, life—and people—are more complicated than that. She started writing about the false growth mindset. In an interview with The Atlantic, Dweck explained it like this:

"False growth mindset is saying you have growth mindset when you don't really have it or you don't really understand what it is. It's also false in the sense that nobody has a growth mindset in everything all the time. Everyone is a mixture of fixed and growth mindsets. You could have a predominant growth mindset in an area but there can still be things that trigger you into a fixed mindset trait. Something really challenging and outside your comfort zone can trigger it, or, if you encounter someone who is much better than you at something you pride yourself on, you can think "Oh, that person has ability, not me." Therefore, I think we all, students and adults, have to look for our fixed-mindset triggers and understand when we are falling into that mindset".

"I think a lot of what happened [with false growth mindset among educators] is that instead of taking this long and difficult journey, where you work on understanding your triggers, working with them, and over time being able to stay in a growth mindset more and more, many educators just said, "Oh yeah, I have a growth mindset" because either they know it's the right mindset to have or they understood it in a way that made it seem easy".

In short, we need to recognize our strengths and our

weaknesses, and be realistic about our talents, passions and opportunities. Yes, you could spend a lot of time becoming proficient at playing the trombone, but is that really where you want to spend your time and energy? With a growth mindset, it's one thing to recognize that you have the potential to learn and develop a set of skills, but it is another to follow that particular path. That's where passion and purpose come into play. Without them, you are not very likely to have the energy and drive needed to become proficient, let alone master, a specific talent.

The growth mindset, however, is still incredibly powerful. It means that developing a talent that is meaningful to you is always possible. And charismatic people teach and demonstrate that inspirational and empowering way of thinking—about anything.

The takeaway about mindset is that anything is possible, if you put your mind and heart to it. And your message is that, as a charismatic figure, you have applied it in your own life, overcoming obstacles along the way to achieve success.

If you are going to be charismatic, people need to warm to you. They must identify with you, and you must identify with them. Your stories must show that, despite whatever perceived status you might have, you recognize and understand the challenges of life and how to overcome them. That is the first step in truly empowering others.

Developing Charisma 4: Appearance

I have already explained the major role of non-verbal communication in perception. Posture, facial expression and gesture all provide visual cues which have associated, often subconscious meanings. And the same goes for your appearance in general. Every aspect of how you look impacts perception, consciously or otherwise.

When I talk about appearance, your first thought might have automatically gone to clothes. Clothes are definitely important, but appearance is way more than what you are wearing.

Have you ever looked at a guy you didn't know and thought *he seems like a nice man*? For all you know, he might be serial killer, a terrorist or a demonic maniac, but based on your first impression, he seems to be a nice man.

What makes you think he's a nice guy? The kind smile he has on his face? The humble expression and posture he exudes? The fact that he let someone in front of him in the checkout aisle or held the door open for the person behind him? Or the fact that he was wearing glasses?

Let's use wearing glasses as an example of the effects of

appearance. There has been research suggesting that people who wear glasses are seen as smarter and more competent. In fact, it is generally accepted that, absent any information about intelligence and competence, wearing spectacles improves your perceived intelligence. However, it is important to recognize that there may be situations where intelligence and competence aren't perceived as the most important characteristics. For example, one study showed that in times of crisis, not wearing spectacles somehow connoted dominance which was deemed a very valuable asset in a crisis situation.

There's also the possibility that wearing glasses is associated with aging and even ill health. In an interesting spin on this topic, genetic researchers from the University of Edinburgh concluded that those people who actually need glasses are 30% more likely to have a high IQ than those who don't. So, if the need to appear smart is a high priority, try non-prescription glasses.

"Everybody knows that intelligence and education are very highly correlated. What they don't know is that physical attractiveness is as equally highly correlated with intelligence as education is. If you want to estimate someone's intelligence without giving them an IQ test, you would do just as well to base your estimate on their physical attractiveness as you would to base it on their years of education," says Kanazawa.

Well put together people, attractive people, are often seen to be more effective in communication and to wield more influence, thus tend to have better success in jobs that involve interfacing with others. For example, less attractive quarterbacks in the NFL make 6% less than their more handsome and equally capable counterparts. (Come to think of it, I can't remember an ugly quarterback.)

Studies on attractiveness generally seem to involve people who are classically attractive, with specific facial dimensions and characteristics. However, any of us can be seen as attractive, even beautiful, and thus elicit the same positive feelings as those who fall into the classical beauty definition.

Attractiveness is, a big deal, No, a huge deal. It is important to make yourself as attractive as possible. This could mean anything from exaggerating your best features to wearing clothes that compliment your body type.

No matter how good your natural appearance is, it is enhanced by the right tone of voice, posture, gestures and message.

This raises the important point that you need to consider what are the most important attributes you want to convey. Perhaps intelligence is key in which case you might decide to sacrifice some perceived attractiveness to ensure that you are seen as smart by wearing those readers.

The first impression is critical. This is the anchoring bias where a first impression tends to anchor subsequent perceptions. It anchors the perceptions that someone has about you, and it is difficult to change them. We use the confirmation bias to confirm our views. So, if you are initially seen as smart and delightful, you have to really screw up to change that perception. Alternatively, if you are initially seen as an untidy idiot, you're going to have to work very, very hard to change that perception.

As far as clothes are concerned, they can go a long way to sculpting our first and following perceptions. Fashion aficionados will consciously focus on how you dress, while others might be more subconsciously influenced.

Your clothes need to highlight your physical strong points

and be appropriate for the occasion. So, if you are carrying a bit too much weight, don't show up in striped clothes that accentuate your girth, unless you're giving a talk on fat- shaming or the problems of the obese. Obviously, context is critical. It makes sense for President Trump to show up at a political rally wearing a Trump hat, but it wouldn't be appropriate if he were attending a funeral. Understand the context you are going to be in, and the audience and their expectations. You can't afford to get that wrong.

I have a true funny story about getting the context completely wrong.

It involves the brother of a friend of mine, Mike, who moves in pretty aristocratic social circles. He was invited to a costume party where the theme was food. After thinking long and hard about the costume he would wear he had the brilliant idea of reaching out to an acquaintance who was connected to some theatrical costumiers. He duly went along to the costumiers and was delighted to find the perfect outfit—a potato! When the day came, he donned his costume and drove to the mansion where the party was to be held.

He marched up the steps and rang the bell. The butler duly answered, and after looking at Mike with a confused expression, he duly announced the potato to the rest of the guests, who were all looking glamorous in their usual formal wear. Poor Mike! He had got the wrong date! It's important to remember that even if you get the dress code wrong, you must always walk with your head up high with a great attitude. Just watch: your friends will be laughing *with* you rather than *at* you.

Posture is very important. Have you ever seen photos of people in the early part of the twentieth century, a hundred years ago? Ladies are walking with heads held high as are the men who more often than not are in top hats. You can't wear a top hat if you're slouching as we do today after years of sitting at desks and poring over computer screens. A hunched or slumped posture looks like defeat. It connotes someone who is carrying a heavy burden that they cannot effectively manage. On the contrary, an erect posture implies someone who is upright and in control. People who stand up tall are straight, not crooked.

Facial gestures amplify your words and intentions. They convey your energy, commitment and passion. Your smile radiates your compassion, understanding and even your sense of adventure.

Your eye-contact reflects your degree of openness and ability to listen when talking. Think about it. People who can't look you in the eye are either afraid or have something to hide.

Speak clearly. This not only makes it easier to hear you, but shows that you possess clarity. Clarity of purpose and clarity of mind. Think about someone who mumbles. Do they have something to hide? Are they ambiguous about what they want to say? Do they even know what they want to say? Or perhaps they are drunk, on drugs, or literally losing their minds?

Pauses can be used to give listeners time to think about what you have just said. Keeping them waiting for what will come out of your mouth next. However, if you pause too long, your audience will wonder if you have forgotten what you want to say or are confused.

list them difficult things to do, they just take practice. You can practice them in front of a mirror, or better yet, into a camera. Making videos of yourself is now so easy that this is probably the best way of practicing your overall appearance.

You will be able to see the improvement as you practice. And taking your practice into real life situations will give you great feedback about how others respond to you.

Developing Charisma 5: Emotional Intelligence

We read all the time that one of the most important characteristics for a leader to have is emotional intelligence. Instinctively, we might think that the term is an oxymoron, because emotions and intelligence are two quite different things So, just what is emotional intelligence?

A simple view of the brain divides it into what is often called the primitive brain and then higher consciousness. Indeed, you can actually see how those structures are organized within the brain, with the lower areas mostly associated with primitive needs, including emotions, and the newly developed areas, the cortical areas, at the top related to consciousness and reasoning.

However, dividing these two functions and thinking of them as separate and distinct parts of the brain is a mistake. They are incredibly interconnected and understanding how that interconnection manifests itself in our feelings, thoughts and actions, and managing it effectively, is what emotional intelligence is all about.

The primitive brain is built around the need for survival. It has all the basic physical functions like breathing, and an alert system to tell us when we're in danger. The primitive brain's main goal is survival. When we're in trouble, the alarm goes off. Lots of things happen within the body to help us deal with the threat but in the mind, the alarms come in the form of emotions.

Emotions alert us to change, something we need to pay attention to. They are the conscious byproducts of physical changes set off by the alarm system.

You may think that I am talking about "negative" emotions. However, there's no such thing as a negative emotion. Emotions are designed to help you pay attention. Although alarms might signal that something bad is going to happen, they are not inherently "negative". Feeling the alarm might be very uncomfortable but don't blame the messenger. Be grateful that you have a good alarm system in place.

Understanding what the alarm is signaling is at the core of emotional intelligence. Many of us confuse feeling the alarm with the difficulty we now have to face. Just feeling the alarm causes you to start feeling anxious. Most of the time you know why the anxiety alarm has been set off. You are losing control of a situation; you're not going to get that important project done in time; you think you're about to lose your job; you think you're about to be exposed in some painful way. Your mind starts racing, and a tsunami of emotion is surging through your body causing you to realize you have to turn the alarm off and NOW!

You race to the drinks' cabinet, or to the refrigerator, or the medicine cabinet, or all three. You must shut off that damn alarm!! While that alarm is pounding through your body, your mind is responding with racing thoughts, creating all sorts of exaggerated scenarios. The emotion crushes any rational thinking and fills your consciousness with horrible thoughts and images as you collapse under the weight of the onslaught. This drives you inevitably to more eating, drinking and medication to turn that shrieking alarm off. And the more you try to turn it off, the louder it gets.

It doesn't have to be that way. Suppose you did something different.

The alarm goes off and that energy starts to flood your mind and body. However, you know it's just an alarm. When you understand how it works, you know how to control the initial energy surge. You know that slow controlled breathing, will slow down the fight/fight system. You also know that the main role of the stress response is to give you energy to run or fight. However, this isn't a physical threat and you don't need all that energy. You know you must move to expend some of that extra energy: go for a walk or just move to burn it off.

You also become aware that your consciousness is under attack and you can't let the feelings overwhelm your mind. If they do, you'll be in big trouble, because any rational thinking will be swallowed up by your fear. Relax. Focus on the present. Listen to your breath and breathe deeply. The deeper and more even your breath, the calmer you will become. This is meditation in action. You become more mindful. Make it a game to turn negative thoughts into positive ones and watch as the tsunami turns from a tidal wave into a trickle. With the alarm turned off, you can now focus on dealing with the challenge that started the whole process off. How realistic is your assessment? How severe is the threat? What plans of action could you create that would manage the apparent problem? Who can you get to help you with these plans? When you can ask these questions, you are on your way to solving the problem, and practicing the development of one of life's most important skills: your resilience.

A IS FOR ADAPTATION

The person who can identify and manage their emotions effectively is at least one step ahead of everyone else. They are in control.

Who would you be inspired by more? A boss who flips out whenever there is a problem, or one who acknowledges the challenge, inspires you to remain calm and helps create a list of solutions?

Charismatic people don't panic. When you can identify emotions and aren't terrified by them, you can meet them head on. And you also become very adept at understanding other people's emotional states and their ways of coping with them. This is a huge advantage, especially in communication and in managing relationships.

So far, I have been talking about uncomfortable emotions but what about the comfortable ones like, joy or pleasure? Surely, we think of charismatic people as energized not dull and unemotional?

Feeling out of control is one of the essential elements of stress. Imagine the power you would have if you had emotional mastery, especially when others are giving in to their feelings. There's a famous Rudyard Kipling poem, "If," that speaks to this subject:

If you can keep your head when all about you
Are losing theirs and blaming it on you,
If you can trust yourself when all men doubt you,
But make allowance for their doubting too;
If you can wait and not be tired by waiting,
Or being lied about, don't deal in lies,
Or being hated, don't give way to hating,
And yet don't look too good, nor talk too wise:
If you can dream—and not make dreams your master;
If you can think—and not make thoughts your aim;
If you can meet with Triumph and Disaster
And treat those two impostors just the same;
If you can bear to hear the truth you've spoken
Twisted by knaves to make a trap for fools,
Or watch the things you gave your life to, broken,
And stoop and build'em up with worn-out tools:
If you can make one heap of all your winnings
And risk it on one turn of pitch-and-toss,
And lose, and start again at your beginnings
And never breathe a word about your loss;
If you can force your heart and nerve and sinew
To serve your turn long after they are gone,
And so hold on when there is nothing in you
Except the Will which says to them:
'Hold on!'
If you can talk with crowds and keep your virtue,
Or walk with Kings—nor lose the common touch,
If neither foes nor loving friends can hurt you,
If all men count with you, but none too much;
If you can fill the unforgiving minute

With sixty seconds' worth of distance run,
Yours is the Earth and everything that's in it,
And—which is more—you'll be a Man, my son!

Emotional intelligence then is about the ultimate control. It's not avoidance, it's adaptation of the greatest kind. It's the ultimate control of the mind. And not just yours.

Suppose someone you know is struggling emotionally. They are very stressed. What is being communicated if you say: "C'mon! Just pull yourself together!"

Apart from being ineffective, it also implies that you can't handle the emotions you feel from seeing someone else be emotional.

What is being communicated if you calmly ask them: "What is going through your mind right now?"

Apart from validating their feeling, you are modeling emotional control. The feeling they have is important, but they can control it.

Pretending you don't have the feeling is not the answer. Recognizing the feeling and knowing you have the ability to actually do something about it is very empowering.

Admitting to feelings is fine; showing that you can deal with them effectively is even better.

Charismatic people channel their emotions. They have control over them to the point where they can use them to communicate very effectively. Control over their emotions is one of the key features of charismatic people that shows people that they can control their emotions and elicit an emotional response in others.

Emotions are linked to memory. The greater the emotion, especially uplifting emotion, the stronger the memory. Uncomfortable emotions work like that, too, with greater discomfort leading to more ingrained memories. Very uncomfortable emotions can reach a point when they actually suppress the memory. The key takeaway is that if you make someone feel good, they will remember the encounter and they will certainly remember you. When you have created a positive association in someone's mind, they will very often exaggerate that feeling and use the "halo effect" to attribute all sorts of amazing attributes to you.

Emotions are also linked to perception. If you are feeling grumpy, depressed, or anxious, those moods will influence how you interpret the things that are going on around you. They will also influence your thoughts. If the person in the next cubicle is laughing and conveying energy and passion your mood will likely determine your perception. When you're in a "good" mood, her laugh will be uplifting and precious, when you're grumpy it will be annoying and disruptive.

So, emotional intelligence isn't just about how you feel, it's also about how you think.

There are numerous paths to successful emotional intelligence.

The first is to understand the role of emotions and the precious skill of recognizing and managing them.

It's also useful to understand the principle that underpin many emotions:

- Anger comes from the perception that you have been treated unfairly
- Stress comes from the perception of being out of control
- Guilt comes from the perception that you have violated some moral principle that is important to you.

- Frustration comes on the perception of being blocked or thwarted.
- Passion comes from the perception that you are manifesting your purpose

The second principle is to practice good physical "relaxation" skills, like controlled breathing that can manage the physical changes that occur with many emotional states.

The third is to practice control of your consciousness, that allows you to recognize feelings but keep them under control. Mindfulness and meditation techniques are great at training your brain to do just that: recognize the moment but not get overwhelmed by it.

Emotional intelligence is therefore an essential part of charisma, allowing you to manage yourself and influence others.

Developing Charisma 6: Healthy Lifestyles

Charisma is about your energy, and energy is the key to wellness. I stressed throughout this book that a healthy lifestyle gives you the energy needed to be charismatic.

There are many elements to a healthy lifestyle that give you energy, but the five key ones are: nutrition, exercise, stress management, sleep and stimulation.

NUTRITION

Nutrition is more than just food, it is the basis of your physiological state, providing the chemical building blocks of both your brain and body. And what you eat is directly related to your energy levels. We also now understand the importance of the microbiome, an environment of millions of bacteria in the gut that impacts not just your physical health but mental health, too. For example, neurotransmitters like serotonin are made in the gut.

Foods that are high in sugar, the so-called high glycemic foods, increase your blood glucose, giving you a rush of energy.

However, as those blood-sugar levels rapidly fall, you will feel tired and lethargic. This might prompt you to eat more, or take a nap. Therefore, high glycemic sugary foods are very poor for your energy levels.

I am convinced that the healthiest diet is a plant-based one. Eating natural plant-based food is far, far healthier than a lot of processed food with a lot of preservatives. The science is pretty clear that a plant-based diet is the healthiest for human beings.

I have been an active animal advocate since I was a child, and veganism is fundamental to my life's journey. I believe in the principle of ahimsa and living as cruelty free as possible. I think that by doing so, we create better karma and in turn build stronger charisma.

EXERCISE

The best stress manager and energizer is physical movement. If charisma is about energy, then exercise has to be part of your life. In addition to keeping you in good if not great physical shape, it also aids learning. There are several studies that show for example that. Aerobically fit kids do better on academic tests.

The current recommendations call for 150 minutes a week of moderate intensity which could be walking, biking, swimming, pretty much anything that gets you up and moving. Or half of that, about 75 minutes of more vigorous exercise. More than either of those two times seem to confer more advantages.

In addition, the President's Council on Sports, Fitness and Nutrition recommends muscle-strengthening exercises, with doing muscle-strengthening activities of moderate or greater intensity that involve all major muscle groups on 2 or more days a week.

Physical activity must be a regular part of your lifestyle. Things that can help you get started if you're not already there are:

- **Choose an activity that you like doing**. If you don't like doing any physical activity, make it enjoyable by listening to your favorite playlists, audiobooks, or other material.
- **Go on walks with friends or family**. And don't just walk; chat, have a good time as you exercise. Engaging friends to exercise with not only makes it more enjoyable it will hold you more accountable.
- **Exercise in nature so you can enjoy natural peace and beauty**. Immersing yourself in these other experiences will not only make exercising more fun, you will find that you can move more easily. The focus doesn't have to be on your movement when you move, it can be on the experience of your social and physical surroundings.
- **Start off with manageable distances and increase them gradually**. I have a friend who was an adamant non-exerciser. She was eventually convinced to walk to her mailbox and back. She gradually increased her distances and ended up being a competitive race-walker!

Physical exercise has so many values, it simply can't be ignored. We are made to move and when we do, we become energized physically and mentally.

STRESS MANAGEMENT

Stress is a major health buster. How can you show charisma if you can't demonstrate emotional control even under difficult circumstances? How can you inspire others if you can't show how you successfully deal with your own life struggles? And prolonged stress is related to the risk of getting almost any of the major illnesses. Stress severely impacts the immune system, rendering you very vulnerable. You need to be healthy and vibrant to be charismatic.

Simple stress management strategies include slow, controlled deep breathing that slows down the stress response, as well as mindfulness exercises in which you switch off mental processing and allow yourself to just experience the moment rather than judging or interpreting it.

And as mentioned above, regular physical activity uses up the excess energy created by the stress response which is, after all, designed to help you run and fight.

SLEEP

Sleep is another critical function. While your brain doesn't actually fall asleep it sends you to sleep so it can carry out two very important functions: clearing your brain of toxins and waste, and consolidating your memories and what you have learned during the previous day.

The first task, waste clearance from the brain, is linked to cognitive decline and dementia. Poor sleep doesn't allow those toxins to be removed creating a dangerous accumulation of waste.

Consolidating your memories and integrating them into your brain and mind is also essential. Learning changes the brain, but poor sleep inhibits that learning process. This happens during the REM stage: dreaming sleep.

It's difficult to be charismatic and sleepy at the same time. It's difficult to be charismatic and not be mentally active, continuing to learn and grow.

There are some simple steps towards good sleep habits:

- Reduce the level of stimulation for an hour or so before going to sleep. For example, you might relax in bed reading or do some simple puzzles. Keep illumination turned down and the room, at a fairly cool temperature, ideally with the window open.
- Go to sleep at the same time and try to get up at the same time. Your body will adjust to these habits.
- Keep the bedroom for relaxation and intimacy. Ideally minimize technologies, like TVs and computers.
- Don't eat for at least two hours before going to bed. The digestive process can interfere with your sleep.
- Alcohol does not improve your sleep. It might make you sleepy but typically it wakes you up before you get into the critical stages of sleep, thus badly interrupting the positive benefits of sleep.
- Ideally, no caffeine, including chocolate, for several hours before your sleep time.

Various fitness trackers allow sleep to be tracked and often divided into the key stages: light, REM (dreaming sleep) and Slow wave deep sleep.

COGNITIVE AND SOCIAL STIMULATION

The brain is energized and grows through stimulation. If you want to be a charismatic person who stimulates others, you must keep yourself stimulated. This means challenging yourself with tasks that push your limits and help you learn new skills.

Similarly, social stimulation is key for the charismatic person, because that is the context in which they spread their energy and vibe. Challenge is the key to growth. While doing crosswords and playing sudoku might be fun, the activities that help you grow are really challenging ones like learning a language or playing an instrument. Think how charismatic it is to be able to converse in several languages, or to be able to sit at a keyboard and play some delightful music.

Think of ways you can challenge yourself. What would you like to be able to do that you can't do now, that would enhance your self-acceptance and inspire the admiration of others?

All of these five behaviors; nutrition, exercise, stress management, sleep and stimulation will not just keep you healthy, but also increase your energy and your ability to influence and inspire others.

Developing Charisma 7: Virtues

The underpinnings of charisma are based in virtues, which when followed naturally and authentically, automatically give you a charismatic demeanor.

Compassion will not only drive you to help others, it will enable them to see you as a caring person. Compassion means supporting people through understanding their situation and empowering them to adapt and overcome their problems.

Compassion is developed when you are able to get outside the egotistical limits of perception and simply allow yourself to experience. This is achieved through mindfulness exercises and meditation. During a study conducted by Harvard Medical School neuroscientist Sara Lazar, researchers looked at experienced meditators and compared them to a control group, including MRI scans of their brains. They were shown not only to develop more compassion but other virtues too. And there was also evidence that experienced meditators had changed the structure of their brains making them more mindful and more emotionally intelligent.

Gratitude will reflect a charismatic grace and keep you

balanced emotionally, especially at times of difficulty where it is easy to look at the negative rather than the positive, what you don't have rather than what you do have.

Gratitude is a mindset. Each day remind yourself of the things in life you are grateful for. Imagine people around the world who don't have the advantages that you have, like a roof over their heads, food, family, relationships, stability, etc.

Forgiveness of both yourself and others will help you from being trapped in the past and allow you to focus on adaptive, resilient and very positive behaviors.

Forgiveness is as much about freeing yourself as it is freeing others. Are there things that you have done in life that you have yet to forgive yourself for? If so, work on those first. Forgiveness is not a free pass, but an acceptance of action. The recognition that it hurt someone else, and acknowledgement that you won't do that again.

Humility will allow others to see you as a warm person rather than just an egotist. It will allow you to connect authentically with people.

Humility is simply recognizing that you are not the center of the universe, and trying the balance between being successful in an egotistical culture, and the recognition that we are interdependent, not just independent. As Rick Warren says, "Humility isn't thinking less of yourself, it's thinking of yourself less".

Acceptance not only will make you seem more positive and approachable, but will help you during difficult times, to remain calm and solve problems.

Acceptance is a crucial part of adaptation and thus charisma. Are there things that you have not accepted about your life? Perhaps you are in denial about your marriage, relationships, career, passion, meaning and life and haven't accepted the reality of where you are.

Respect of others will elicit people's respect of you. It's very easy in today's culture to violently oppose points of view that differ from yours, but while that might get a lot of views, it won't win people over or elicit respect.

Respect is based on an open-mindedness that allows you to step aside from your own views and emotions and try to understand where another person is coming from. Understanding is not the same as agreeing or endorsing or even tolerating.

Nonjudgement, another virtue which is increasingly difficult to adopt as a personal attribute in a social media environment where people are increasingly becoming extreme in their views.

Being nonjudgmental allows you to listen seriously and try to fully understand what the other person is saying and why they believe what they do. In a mindful way, don't presume and attribute ideas to the other person that they have not expressed. You want to be heard and not judged, so act towards others the way you want them to act with you. You can develop your respect of other people by first recognizing that as human beings you have way more in common than you think. Recognize that if you had the same life experiences, you might very well think the same way.

Altruism is a key to charisma, allowing you to go beyond yourself, into something greater, also known as self-transcendence.

Altruism can be developed by volunteering for a charitable cause, which will have benefits for you as well as the beneficiary of your efforts. Do you volunteer for such a venture? If not, start doing so by researching local opportunities and volunteering for one or more of them.

Courage is a virtue. It allows you to remain authentic and accepting without fleeing because of fear. You can't very easily be charismatic if you are a coward. Not that fear isn't real, it is, but you need to prevent it from becoming a handicap in your development.

Courage can be developed simply by facing up honestly to whatever situation you are facing. When you face your issues honestly and with courage they often don't seem to be as problematic, because you are not hiding the truth.

Honesty is critical. If you're dishonest with others you are also likely to be dishonest with yourself, a recipe for disaster which will prevent you from being very effective at adopting many of the charisma skills and characteristics.

Honesty is having the courage to face the reality of your situation. Lying, especially to yourself, prevents you from adequately accepting what is in front of you. It's often a temporary reaction that prolongs the problem.

Patience is very definitely a virtue and is a sign of emotional control. It can be enhanced by mindfulness and meditation and is critical if you want to make considered and thoughtful decisions rather than impulsive choices.

Patience is a skill that you can develop and practice. It requires you to take time to really consider or enact decisions. Even if you instantly know the answer to an issue, still give yourself time to fully consider all the alternatives and think through the possible outcomes.

These virtues interact with each other to provide an authentic, emotionally intelligent compassionate person who rightly elicits praise and acclaim, especially in an increasingly divided world.

References

Dweck, C. (2006) Mindset: The New Psychology of Success. Random House.

Hill, W. D., et al. (2018) "A combined analysis of genetically correlated traits identifies 187 loci and a role for neurogenesis and myelination in intelligence." Molecular Psychiatry volume 24, pages169–181(2019)

Mehrabian, Albert & Wiener, Morton (1967). "Decoding of Inconsistent Communications". Journal of Personality and Social Psychology.

Mischel, W., Shoda, Y., & Rodriguez, M. L. (1989). Delay of gratification in children. Science, 244, 933–938.

Prochaska, J. O., & DiClemente, C. C. (1983). Stages and processes of self-change of smoking: Toward an integrative model of change. Journal of Consulting and Clinical Psychology, 51(3), 390–395.

Rogers, P. & Wiseman, R. (2006) Self-perceived high intuitiveness: An initial exploration. Imagination, Cognition & Personality, 25(2), 161-177.